Comments

"The exact same thing happened to our family."

"I cried when I read it."

"We have to talk about it, even though it's hard sometimes."

"It made me think of my dad."

"So many people will be able to relate to this topic."

"Our family is still in a mess."

"When we lost our mom, things were never the same for our family."

"This book will help people to see things differently."

"It's an unfortunate reality."

I
REM*
MB*R

Nikki,

I hope you enjoy reading this book as much as I have enjoyed writing it. Thank you for your support!

Vanessa K Williams Harvey

Publisher Page

Vanessa K. Williams-Harvey

Acknowledgements

I would like to thank my family and especially my husband Mark, for encouragement and support in sharing this message with the world. Your unwavering sincerity has fueled a desire to strive for positives when negativity is all around.

I would also like to thank my friends, colleagues and siblings for joining me on this ride. Your continued acceptance and appreciation mean more to me than you will ever know.

I would be remiss if I did not thank my dear Mother, whose impact on my life continues to be the driving force that allows me to awaken each day with the goal of doing more, being more and reaching for more--while I can.

To the Family Unit, whatever or whomever that may look like for you!

Jeremiah 29:11

"For I know the plans I have for you," declares the Lord, "plans to prosper you and not to harm you, plans to give you hope and a future."

Contents

Chapter 1	*The Lake*
Chapter 2	*The Projects*
Chapter 3	*The Bank*
Chapter 4	*The Little Blue Pill*
Chapter 5	*The Beauty Shop*
Chapter 6	*The Evaluation*
Chapter 7	*The Restaurant*
Chapter 8	*The Light*
Chapter 9	*The Church*
Chapter 10	*The Decision*
Chapter 11	*The Visit*
Chapter 12	*The Café*
Chapter 13	*The Reflection*
Chapter 14	*The Change*

Chapter 1

I Remember ... *the Lake*

It was late in the afternoon of a crisp, fall day when my home phone rang. Noticing Mother's name on the caller ID, I casually picked up the receiver to see what was going on. It was normal for Mother and me to chat on the phone every day, even if we did not have much to talk about. Mostly I would call to say, "What are you doing?" and Mother would sigh because she knew I really didn't want anything; I was just calling to check in. When we chatted, we typically talked mostly about nothing. Mother was about 68 years old and mostly retired. She worked when she wanted but mostly seemed to enjoy her life as it was. Our daily phone call was an opportunity for me to check up on her and to make sure everything was okay.

This particular call was a bit odd, although at first it seemed like no big deal. Mother calmly said, "I cannot find the place." "OK," I said. "What place are you talking about?" She explained that she had found a coupon in the mail for a manicure at a particular nail salon. Since this nail salon was new in town and Mother had never been there before, I wasn't surprised that she couldn't find it.

"Where is this place located?" I asked. Mother replied, "It's on Taylorsville Road." That didn't tell me much, because Taylorville Road is a long, heavily traveled road that stretches from the bustling city streets of Louisville to a quiet, desolate country-like setting near Taylorsville Lake. When I asked her where the salon was on Taylorsville Road, her reply baffled me. "I'm headed towards Taylorsville Lake," she said. I paused for a minute and tried to envision exactly where Mother was and where it was she should have been headed.

Nothing was making much sense at this point, but I didn't want to rush to judgment. Mother had never made me feel uncomfortable about her actions, but she obviously needed help or she wouldn't have called in the first place. At that point, I awkwardly asked her for the address of the nail salon she was trying to find and told her to pull over to the side of the road so that she could read the address and telephone number off the coupon. I jotted the address down on a napkin, then asked her to read off the address of where she was parked. She was able to give me the numbers off a mailbox, and that confirmed that she had driven out too far and had passed her destination. I kept her on the home phone while I called the nail salon on my cellphone. I was able to reach someone at the nail salon, confirm the address, and get a landmark and cross street. Once I knew the exact location of the nail salon, I hung up my cellphone and resumed my conversation with Mother.

I told her that I had the directions of the nail salon and that she needed to turn her car around and drive in the opposite direction. My voice raised a pitch or two higher when she still questioned which direction to drive and I blurted out, "Drive away from Taylorsville Lake. Drive towards town!" I went on to explain that the nail salon was in the shopping center on Taylorsville Road with the big bowling alley right out front.

Then, the conversation got weird. Mother didn't want me to be alarmed, but she clearly knew something was wrong or she would not have called in the first place. Our conversation went something like this:

> Me: "Where are you?"
> Mother: "I don't know."
> Me: "Do you see the shopping center?"

Mother: "I don't see anything."
Me: "What does the street sign say?"
Mother: "Taylorsville Lake." (At this point, my heart started to pump faster, because nothing she said sounded right.)
Me: "Does anything look familiar?"
Mother: "NO!"
Me: "You need to turn around now!"

Somewhat alarmed, I told my husband, Mike, "We need to go make sure Mother is where she is supposed to be." This was something new to us and so very different.

Mother had always been extremely fearless and independent. It was not at all like her to get turned around. After decades of driving us all around the streets of Louisville, she knew the community like the back of her hand. It was very odd for her not to know how to get to the nail salon when given the address.

She must have heard the urgency in my voice when I told her to drive toward town and away from Taylorsville Lake because she turned her car around and started heading in the opposite direction. With her finally headed the right way, I transferred the call to my cellphone, and Mike and I got in our car to go meet her.

As Mike drove, I stayed in contact with Mother. (Yes, I know that she probably shouldn't have been driving and talking on her cellphone, but we had no other choice.) I told her to call out the landmarks she passed as she drove back into town. She said, "I'm passing under the expressway," which was a good sign if she was going in the right direction. "Now, I'm passing Watterson

Expressway," she said next. That was music to my ears, because things were making sense now.

I asked Mother about particular landmarks that had always been easily known to her but that now seemed unfamiliar. I said, "You'll be coming up on the shopping center in about a mile. It will be on your right-hand side near the bowling alley." "I know where that is," she replied. I was so relieved that she was familiar with what I was saying.

By the time Mike and I arrived at the nail salon, there sat Mother smiling and having a manicure as if nothing unusual had happened. The three of us looked at each other and shook our heads searching for understanding. Mother sort of laughed at herself and actually had the nerve to ask us what we were doing there. I told her that we had to make sure she was able to find the nail salon.

Mike and I sat in the nail salon and watched Mother for a while. The nail technician got a kick out of our tale about Mother's adventurous journey down Taylorsville Road. I think it made Mike and I feel better to see Mother smiling widely because, in our minds, she was where she was supposed to be. She kept telling us that we could leave. We chatted with her and gave her our own little test to see if she was "with it." She laughed it off and assured us that we could go on home and that she would be fine.

Mike and I left, not saying much during what seemed to be a long ten-minute drive to our house. It was one of those situations where you are so enthralled with your thoughts that you can't recall how you got from point A to point B and remember nothing in between. I think everyone had a lot on their minds after that day.

I shook my head in disbelief and wondered to myself what in the world had just happened. If I had not told Mother to turn around when I did, I have no idea where she would have ended up. Thank God for divine intervention. Everything ended on a good note. Mother was where she intended to be, and we had made sure of that. We really didn't think much of it and really didn't give it much thought. We figure, Mother simply took the scenic route to the nail salon ... or so we thought. I felt so much better because the situation was not as bad as I initially thought.

  Later that evening, I called Mother to check up on her. She answered the phone after two or three rings. If I timed it just right, I could catch her before her nightly news programs came on television. My siblings and I had learned that if we disturbed her during one of her shows we would have to listen to her reprimand us as if we were children. Yes, we were her children but I was forty-four at the time. I must have timed it just right, because Mother answered the phone casually. I asked her how she was doing and she replied, "Girl, I am fine," followed by a slight giggle. How I wish that were true.

  She was fine, at least for now. I felt comforted in hearing her say this. Little did I know that a thief called Alzheimer's disease was knocking at her front door.

Chapter 2

I Remember ... *the Projects*

All my life, Mother was the queen of our castle. We learned early on that it was Mother's way or no way. She was the centerpiece and rock-solid foundation for our family.

As with all families, we had our fair share of drama and disagreements. There were many times when, were it not for the strength and determination of Mother, our very essence as individuals and as a family unit would have been in grave jeopardy. We all could count on Mother to put the pieces back together, build us up, and tear us down as only a mother could do.

I happen to be the youngest of Mother's five children. Mother married her childhood sweetheart, Sammy Willis, when she was just sixteen years old. At least, that's what we assume since Felicia, my oldest sister, is sixteen and a half years younger than Mother. Some of the dates are a bit fuzzy because for some reason, people either didn't understand the importance of accurate recordkeeping, didn't care or they simply made things up. And, then there were the things that you just did not question or talk about in the family, things children were expected to accept even if we did not fully understand.

We certainly didn't ever discuss Mother's ex-husband, Sammy. After Mother married Sammy, she immediately gave birth in rapid succession, and the young couple soon had three small children to raise, Felicia, Vance, and Shonie. Sammy served in the Army, and the young family settled in Louisville, Kentucky, after moving from Louisiana.

As soon as Sammy moved the family to their new life and away from family support, he showed his true colors. While Mother was tending to her young children in a new city, Sammy was tending to everything else except his family. Once he left us, we didn't ever mention his name. Mother only mentioned him when she would occasionally talk about our no-good fathers. But we all knew what Sammy was, and I vaguely recall him coming around from time to time. When I was very young, I recall he would pop into our lives for a little while, and then he would be gone again—sort of here today and gone tomorrow. I can count the number of times that Sammy would drop in and out on one hand. There is one particular incident with Sammy that I will never forget.

When I was about five or six years old, I remember hearing a lot of shouting seeing people pushing and shoving in a swarm of commotion. We were just inside the door of our small three-bedroom apartment in the projects where Mother and Sammy were arguing. The neighbors had to intervene and came inside to break things up. My eyes were wide and my head was ball of confusion with all of the yelling and fighting going on around me. I strategically positioned myself on top of our refrigerator so that I could see what was going on. There I sat with a butcher knife in my hand, ready to strike. I think I took that position to at least give me a little advantage and authority, not realizing how ill-equipped I was. In my heart of hearts, I was going to do whatever I could to protect Mother from him.

Sammy had come to the house and was confronting Mother about something. My siblings and I were at home where we were supposed to be. And there I sat ready, with my small, skinny fingers tightly squeezing the wooden handle of a large, shiny butcher knife. The knife was probably as big as I was, but I was determined to protect my family and especially Mother. Who knows why at such a young age I would be inclined to grab a knife with the goal of stabbing someone. I realize now that I was willing to do whatever it took to protect Mother. This inclination must be learned very early and carries on throughout our lives. It has certainly guided me through these last few years.

Mercifully, someone plucked the knife from my small hands and helped me down from atop the refrigerator. My siblings and I were sent to the bedroom and instructed to close the door. We just sat motionless with one another, hoping to hear silence and an end to the conflict. We didn't know what else to do. The police were called, Sammy ended up leaving—for good this time, as I recall. Things must have turned out alright, because I don't remember any ambulances being called or anyone going to jail on that particular occasion. After the police left and the neighbors returned to their homes, Mother slowly opened the bedroom door to let us know that it was okay to come out of the bedroom. No one said or did anything for the rest of the evening. We were shaken but not shattered.

Not surprisingly, Sammy was as inept as a father as he was a husband. He more closely displayed the morals and characteristics of the character in the Temptations song that went like this: "Sammy was a rolling stone. Wherever he laid his hat was his home. And when he died, all he left us was alone."

Unfortunately, that was the same theme for the man who fathered Charlene and me, the youngest of Mother's five children. Our biological father was affectionately known by his nickname, "Black Richard," which was a play on his given name and his dark-chocolate skin color. I remember him as being round and of average height, with very dark skin—almost black. He would've reminded me of a black Santa Claus except he never brought any gifts or shared any cheer. I recall him coming around to visit on occasion, but he didn't do much else.

In fact, the only thing I can recall from Black Richard's visits was his signature hair style—processed curly hair styled like a pimp. It sounds funny and I cringe just thinking about it now, but that was the style back then. That visual is the only thing I remember of the man who helped form me yet did absolutely nothing to support, nurture, or to shape me.

Although we liked Black Richard a lot better than the good-for-nothing Sammy, I'm afraid he wasn't much of a father either. Sure, he stayed around for a bit, but he could never do right by us, his children, or by our mother. The older children would give Black Richard a hard time and tell him that they didn't have to obey him because he wasn't their father. They probably had a hand in chasing him away and making him not want to come back. We all knew better than that, even at our young ages. Many, many years later, I found out that Black Richard had another family of his own the whole time, which explained why he didn't have anything for us.

Both Sammy and Black Richard are dead now. They were dead to me long before their respective demise. I must admit that I didn't shed one tear or go to either of their funerals. I felt nothing. My issues with men today are closely tied to what I experienced as a child as a result of their interactions, or lack thereof, with our family. I had to learn to forgive them, yet I still struggle to forget the hurt and pain they caused.

It's ironic how children pick up on certain things. None of us ever referred to Sammy or Black Richard as daddy or father, not that they deserved such titles. Each of us called them by their first names. On the other hand, we instinctively referred to our mother as "Mama," "Ma," or "Mother," because that is the essence of who she was to us. It is difficult to imagine how Mother ended up with them as mates; she was a much better person than either of them. I actually feel the reason Mother settled with Sammy and then Black Richard is because she was looking for something in a man, and she thought they could fulfill that role for her. They turned out to be the two worst excuses for men—let alone fathers—we could have gotten. It appears Mother was looking for love in all of the wrong places, and what she got was of no use to her or any of us. Unfortunately, they failed her and us miserably. I can only imagine how she must've felt and how easy it would've been for her to simply throw in the towel. I am thankful that God put the will, strength, and courage in her heart to fight for herself and her children.

We lived a simple but fun-loving life growing up in the projects. Although times were tough most of the time, Mother made sure we had most of the things we needed and some of the things we wanted. The projects were a bit different back in the late 1960s and early '70s. Everyone looked out for one another, and families tended to get along and help one another out. There was a lot of borrowing from neighbors for what you didn't have and giving to others what you did have to give. It was nothing for Mother to have one of us run next door for a cup of sugar or some laundry detergent. She would kindly reciprocate when the shoe was on the other foot.

Mother worked long hours doing hard work at the bag plant a few blocks from our apartment. Felicia, being the oldest, would often have to watch the younger children. She was essentially a child watching children, but there was always a neighbor's door to knock on in case of an emergency. And we all knew that if Mother got a bad report about us from school or a neighbor, we would be in big trouble.

Occasionally, Mother made special trips to our elementary school for the sole purpose of whipping us after the teacher had to call her. That was back when it was legal for everyone, including teachers, to whip kids; no one got arrested or got their kids removed from the home. We called it the closed-door treatment" That is where teachers and school administrators would give your parents a room for privacy and, after they closed the door, you would get the crap beaten out of you. The only thing people heard was the child wailing behind the closed door. No one dared to interrupt. When Mother finished whipping us, she made us stop crying prior to opening the door, and we had to pull it all together on the spot. When the door opened, it was as if nothing had ever happened as far as everyone was concerned. It was as if whippings were condoned. The adults banded together so that when a young child got reprimanded at school or in the middle of a department store, the thought behind it was, "Spare the rod you spoil the child," which is in the Bible. There was one sure way to get all of our attention and that was to say, "I'm going to tell your mother."

I remember one day waking up bright and early in the morning. We would start our day early, go outside, and play all day long. I must have been around eight years old because it was in 1972. As we were out running and playing, we noticed a crowd gathering. That meant that there was probably something happening or about to happen, so I ran over to see what the excitement was about. I pushed forward to see what was going on. Everyone was admiring a shiny, new, silver 1972 Chevy Monte Carlo parked on the street in the middle of the projects; people were making a big fuss about the new car that was parked along the uneven, concrete sidewalk. I had no idea what all of the fuss was about. Then, someone said, "That's your Mother's new car!" My eyes lit up. I could hardly believe what I was hearing. After working extra shifts at the bag plant, Mother saved up enough money to buy herself a new car. She no longer had to depend on public transportation. Mother didn't particularly like to depend on anything or anyone.

Mother was so full of surprises. Then again, nothing Mother did really surprised us. If anyone could do anything, it was Mother. We all thought Mother was rich, smart, and beautiful. She had everything, but mostly she had us children, who were her biggest fans. Mother's tenacity and working long hours soon paid off. She was able to save enough money the year I turned nine years old and we were able to move out of the projects and into a nice apartment all the way out in the Okolona neighborhood.

Okolona was a far cry from the projects, and things were very different. Our new apartment was very nice, and there were a lot of white people in the neighborhood—mostly white people, in fact.

We moved from a mostly black, poverty-stricken neighborhood to a mostly white, barely-getting-by neighborhood. Mother continued to work mornings at the bag plant and then headed straight to her second job at Airway's, a local department store. It helped that Airways was located directly in front of our apartment complex. We would on occasion run over to see Mother there if not at home. Having Mother close by was a nice bonus even if she was working.

  Things were going along fine until I, along with a group of friends, got the notion to go to Airways and steal Barbie dolls along with all of the accessories. What were we thinking? Well, we weren't thinking; we were just doing. We got away with it a couple of times. Like most thieves, we got greedy and kept going back for more and more until one dreadful day, we got caught red-handed. Security guards surrounded us, and we were taken into the security office like four little criminals. Our only recourse was to call our parents or, in all of our cases, our parent. That meant we each needed the security guard to call our mothers so that we could get released. Well, I am sure it was a bit awkward for Mother as an employee of Airway's to get a call from security that her child had been caught stealing in the store.

  I had sunk to a new low. Nothing could prepare me for the wrath of Mother. The focused look on her face as she arrived to claim me paled in comparison to the unadulterated beating I got when I got home. To say it was bad is an understatement, as I sincerely believe I got the crap beaten out of me. Although I deserved it, by today's standards, Mother would have been locked up had I had that nerve to call the police. But that was not an option in those days. I still get chills when I think about that day. I was also put on punishment and other harsh things were done to me, and I deserved every single thing.

When Mother said jump, we said, "How high?" We couldn't even look at her the wrong way out of fear we would get popped in the mouth. That was back in the day when disciplining your child did not equate to child abuse. We got smacked around when we needed it. We got whipped with a belt when we needed it. Occasionally, we were whipped with an extension cord—when we needed it.

Mother actually had the nerve to suggest we go pick out a switch so she could whip us. No, we couldn't pick a small, flimsy switch, or else she'd send us back to "get a good one." And while getting your whipping, you were inclined to listen to Mother basically preach to you. It went something like this: "Now I have told you…," "Do what I say…," I told you not to…," "Be still…," "You keep on doing stupid stuff…," "Now let that school have to call me again…," and, my personal favorite, "Ain't nobody gonna help you." It is kind of funny thinking about it now. At the time, it was a very different story. I guess it really wasn't as bad as I once feared. Nothing could beat Mother's love.

It seems we all survived and actually turned out pretty well. Despite our challenges growing up, four of Mother's children went on to earn college degrees, mostly due to her expectations and insistence on higher education. I ended up pursing a nursing career. Her sacrifice and guidance was the deciding factor in our determination to succeed.

Although Mother was pleased with the education we received, she was most proud when she decided to pursue her own GED. I was in my early twenty's when Mother decided to pursue her GED. During this journey with Mother, I was tasked with helping her with homework, which was a bit awkward. I have never been the teacher type so it was a challenge tutoring Mother. She reminded me when I slipped up. Tutoring turned out to be like torture for me. There was something about the concept of fractions that Mother struggled with particularly. I cringed at the thought of homework with Mother, but I didn't have a choice in the matter. I felt obligated to help her with her homework. It paid off, and Mother passed a succession of tests and was finally able to graduate. There was a graduation ceremony one evening at Norse Middle School. All of us were there to support Mother on her special day. As I sat in the audience waiting for the PA announcer to call Mother's name, I thought I caught a glimpse of a faceless image in the crowd. When I took a second look, it was gone. My imagination must've been playing tricks on me. It was as if a thief was trying to steal the joy and happiness we all felt on this day. When the recessional was over, we went home for a family celebration. We finally had another reason to give Mother the praise and honor she so deserved. We meant the world to her, but she was everything to each of us. That was how it always had been and how it always would be.

   As I laid in bed that night, I remember how excited Mother was about her graduation. She was almost as proud of herself as she had been for each of us. The glow in her eyes was mesmerizing. I sensed she felt comfort in practicing what she had been preaching to each of us for years. It made me happy that she was happy. I could now roll over in bed knowing that she could be proud of herself.

One of Mother's favorite sayings I remember was, "You don't need a million bucks to look like a million bucks." Mother surely didn't have a million dollars, but you couldn't tell it by looking at her or how she acted. If anyone could make a dollar out of fifteen cents, it was Mother.

Years later, however, she would face a problem that a million dollars couldn't solve.

Chapter 3

I Remember ... *the Bank*

"Come on, go with me," Mother said one day about seven years ago as she set out on her way to run a few errands. I went along with her more out of obligation. I had a ton of things to do myself. I felt guilty for feeling this way. Mother had sacrificed so much and done without that the very least I could do was go to the bank with her.

Easy enough, right?

I hopped in the car with her, but for some reason she wanted me to drive. I really didn't feel like driving, but I obliged and got into the driver's seat. The bank was a mere two miles down the street. I do not recall our conversation as we went on our way. I sat quietly trying to concentrate on the road as I drove. In typical fashion, Mother did all of the talking, and I would nod in agreement now and then. Only after she expected me to initiate some conversation, she would say, "Can you talk?" I just glanced at her, and then she went off on a tangent about when I needed to talk I didn't say anything and when I need to be quiet, you couldn't get me to shut up. We both laughed at ourselves.

I remember that it seemed like Mother was doing less and less for herself and relying more on us to get things done on her behalf. This was very different coming from a woman who was always on the go and so well put together. It wasn't like Mother to ask anyone for anything. If she did ask for help of some sort, it was because she either could not do it for herself or simply didn't know how. Although I felt obligated to do as Mother asked, I surely didn't want to encourage her dependence on me—or anyone else for that matter. Also, resonating in my ear was the commandment to Honor your Mother. Come to think of it, I couldn't recall a time when I had ever said "no" to Mother when asked to do anything.

Things got really weird really fast. It was odd that Mother asked me to go inside the bank with her, as she typically kept her personal business to herself and her affairs in order. Ordinarily, if she even thought you were watching her count money or looking at her checkbook ledger, she would say, "Don't be trying to count my money." I was really surprised when she asked me to fill out the deposit slip for her.

I said, "Do it yourself." Mother responded, "Do it for me, girl." Again, I hesitantly obliged. Mother wanted a check deposited, so I filled out the deposit slip and handed it to her to give to the bank clerk. I had no reason to be alarmed as Mother told me exactly what her intentions were. I simply filled out the information, stepped back from the counter and watched Mother complete her transaction with the clerk. After leaving the bank, we made a couple more stops before we made our way back to Mother's house.

When we pulled up to the house, she invited me in for a few minutes. I told her that I only had a few minutes and needed to run some errands of my own. I went inside and sat with her for a few minutes in the den. Mother lived with Felicia but had her own space in the basement. I could not resist making a visit to Mother's room where she stored her clothes and accessories. This room was adjacent to the sewing room and was filled with racks and racks of clothes, coats, shoes, boots, jewelry, purses, and anything you could possibly think of. I made a quick visit to the clothes room and picked out a shirt that only Mother would have and a cute bracelet for me to wear later that night.

Mother said, "Now why don't you get your own stuff?" I shot back, "Why would I buy my own stuff when I can wear yours?" Mother just shook her head and replied, "I want my stuff back." I nodded as I exited with the items I had selected. Sometimes I would return Mother's things and sometimes I wouldn't. If it was something she really wanted back, Mother would remind me—constantly. She would then lecture me about having my own money and how I should be doing this or that for her. Although I patiently listened and wait for her to finish, in the end, she would always let me have whatever I wanted.

Looking back, I think that Mother knew something was "different" with her, and I am sure she felt more comfortable knowing that one of us was with her for support. I still didn't think there was anything to be too worried about. This is around the time that technology was booming, and Mother was not a technologically savvy person at all. It only seemed natural for her to need our help from time to time. Mother had a basic flip phone that she carried around with her, but it got to a point that it was almost comical for her to use the device. When the comical aspect became too painful to hear or to watch, I reluctantly discontinued her service. When family members asked why I had cut off the cellphone, it was for the simple fact that she couldn't understand how to use it.

In Mother's glory days, she tended to live a carefree life. After all, she had raised her children and later worked as a successful nanny to some of the prominent families in Louisville. They got the benefit of having a loving extension of our mother to share with their families. Mother was thriving and living the good life by all accounts. Since she had long given up on men, her life was filled with travel, entertainment and fun. It was nothing for her to jump on a plane to Los Angeles to visit her siblings or tag along with us on a family vacation. But her favorite pastime was going to the casino, where she would literally gamble all day and night. The casino was an outlet for her and she enjoyed the slot machines. No one dared question why she spent so much time at the casino because the response would be, "Don't be jealous."

Mother would be proud of her winnings from the casino, and she was a savvy gambler. She was not going to lose a lot of money at once, so she made the most of her time at the casino by playing the penny slots. She would spend hour after hour playing on the same ten dollars that she had come to the casino with. I on the other hand would rather lose all of my money in twenty minutes than waste my time playing on the same ten dollars.

But it wasn't about me; it was about Mother and what she liked to do. At this point in our lives, it was always about Mother. Since she appeared to be happy and enjoying life, who were we to question whatever it was that brought her happiness? Little did we know that Mother indeed was living the last years of the best years of her life. Soon and very soon, all of our lives would change forever. None would change as drastically or quickly as our dear Mother.

In the meantime, we went on with our lives without a care in the world. Each of us had our ups and downs, but the good far outweighed the bad. We had the typical family turmoil that every family goes through, but we always seemed to figure things out. Our biggest family challenge was about to rear its ugly head and test our faith, spirit, and sustainability. This challenge would strike at the very core of our foundation and threaten our resolve. No challenge we had ever faced compared to what was about to happen. This would be the ultimate test of faith.

My siblings and I had children of our own, and they all loved "Moner," as they called Mother. Moner is how they addressed each of her greeting cards, and to this day she is still Moner to them. The nickname came about when I was a teenager and the Valley Girl phenomenon was the latest fad. I immediately started calling her "Mother." Mother's first grandchild tried to copy me but could only muster "Moner." Well, it stuck. Now all the grandkids affectionately refer to Mother as "Moner."

I remember stopping by Mother's house while she was babysitting Felicia's son. I was talking with Mother and heard cursing coming from the next room. There was only the three of us in the house. I looked up at Mother when I heard the cursing again. Mother looked away. I asked if that was my nephew cursing. I again looked at Mother in disbelief and asked her what was going on. I couldn't believe my ears. Mother was only able to shake her head. I thought it odd that Mother did not immediately reprimand him nor did she seem to be particularly surprised by what he was saying. I asked Mother what in the world was going on. Mother told me how, when she was in the middle of watching her favorite soap opera, "The Young and the Restless," the local television station interrupted the show for something happening in the news. Mother said that without thinking she blurted out a few choice words about what she thought of the situation which my nephew overheard and decided to repeat what she said. We both watched as this sweet and innocent little boy nonchalantly cursing at any and everything in sight, including his action figures.

      I looked at Mother and she looked at me as we snickered to ourselves so that he didn't notice. After we regained our composure, we fixed the situation by telling him that it wasn't nice to say those kinds of words. We went on to explain that those were bad words and should not be repeated. Mother and I went into another room to laugh some more. I took great pleasure in reminding Mother that she should probably try to set a better example for the kids, if not for herself. Mother kindly reminded me not to be a smartass. It was a good time to laugh, and we took full advantage of it.

Chapter 4

I Remember... *the Little Blue Pill*

Prior to Mother being sentenced to a life living and struggling with Alzheimer's, she worked intermittently as a nanny for some of the more prominent and just plain good families in town. These families trusted no one except Mother to care for their children and to watch out for their most prized possessions. For each of these families, Mother was treated as a member of their extended family. She was given full rein to mold, groom and raise their children as well as acting as a counselor for their parents as only a mother could. You see, Mother played an integral part in nurturing these families just as she had done for our family. Before too long, these families became an extension of our own family. Our lives became intermingled with the common thread being Mother.

    We all knew not to disturb Mother while "The Young and The Restless" was on because one, she probably wouldn't answer the phone anyway, and two, if she did pick up the phone, you would be greeted with a barrage of questions, such as, "Why do you call me when my show is on" and "You know I like this show; now what do you want?" I would roll my eyes and shake my head while listening since Mother couldn't see me on the other end of the phone. I grew accustomed to the tongue-lashings that rolled out of Mother's mouth so easily and at the flip of a switch.

    If any of us really needed to talk to Mother while her shows were on, our best bet was to call her during the commercial. But our timing had to be almost perfect to complete the call before the commercial break ended. While it could be done, I soon learned it was best to simply wait out the hour until her show went off rather than to disturb her. I cannot remember a worse feeling than making the conscious decision to interrupt her show knowing full well she would be angry.

We learned to live with the tongue lashings and didn't pay them much mind. We also seemed to get over them pretty quickly. It was nothing for Mother to curse one of us out if we really did something stupid. Lord knows she meant no harm. I feel certain that she did it out of love. From this experience, I learned to have an open mind about most things and not to take things so personally. I will admit that some of the things Mother said had a way of cutting to my core. For the life of me, I could not imagine how anyone could say such things. It wasn't until I had children of my own did I understand.

Mother was many things, but she was not perfect. It took me a while to realize that she was the best thing to ever happen to us. It frightens me to think how things may have turned out if I had to put up with half of the stuff she did.

In the early evenings, Mother's time was filled with news shows like CNN, where she listened intently to every word that came out of the correspondents' mouths. Mother would also be busy on her sewing machine, making or mending clothes for some of the many people who knew of her skills as a seamstress. You see, when we were growing up, Mother got the bright idea that it would be more economical for her to make our clothes than to buy clothing for five growing kids. Mother bought herself a sewing machine and taught herself to sew. After a few practice items, we soon had the neatest clothes for some of the poorest kids in our school. Mother got really good at sewing and soon she was taking requests to sew for other people. To this day, I still am able to wear some of the clothes she made almost forty years ago. Some of those outfits will never go out of style.

I regret that when she wanted to teach me how to sew I decided that I didn't like it. This is one of the rare times I wish Mother had made me do something I didn't want to do. I'm not exactly sure how I got out of that one, but I did. Now, as Mother's sewing machine sits in a corner of the basement collecting dust, I've just posted on Facebook a request for someone to make me a pillow of all things. If Mother were still Mother, she would have made that pillow for me in a heartbeat. And, you can bet it would be better than anything money could buy.

Mother now has eight grandchildren who all love her very much—in part because she spoiled each of them at every opportunity she got. You know you are fighting a losing battle when your young children tell you, "Ima tell Moner on you"—and they do! Whatever I did that they felt the need to report, they would run into Mother's house when we pulled into the driveway and proudly provide a report of everything I did that they felt was wrong. Mother would look at me with a demoralizing smirk on her face while soaking up all of their gory details. The boys, all four of them, were quite proud of themselves for telling on me. I didn't confirm or deny anything. Clearly their loyalties rested with Moner.

I let the boys visit with Mother as often as they liked. I particularly appreciated when the boys asked to spend the night with her. I would call Mother and begin the conversation by asking how she was doing. After discussing the events of the day or any new gossip, I would speak up and convey the real reason for my call. The conversation would go something like this:

> Me: *"The boys want to come spend the night."*
> Mother: *"You put them up to it."*
> Me: *"No I didn't. They asked if they could come spend the night with you."*
> Mother (never willing to just say yes): *"Well come on, but feed them before they come. I'm not cooking for nobody. I don't have any kids. Feed your own kids. All those boys. Why they want to spend the night with me anyway? You told them to ask to stay with me. Call me before you come."*

As Mother was saying all of that without taking a breath or giving me the opportunity to respond, I would just listen. When she would finally finish, I would said, "OK. Thanks."

The boys knew that when they went to Mother's it would be just like one big pajama party. They would have full rein of the basement and snacks galore while sleeping on the floor in sleeping bags. There would also be an endless amount of video games and movies and plenty of room for horseplay. I appreciated Mother helping with the boys and was thankful for the opportunity for Mike and me to spend some quality time together.

I made it a point to try to pick the boys up early following sleepovers at Mother's, but occasionally I would be later than originally planned. Needless to say, she would call to wake me up and remind me to "Come and get these boys." There would be no greeting at all. She didn't care how I was doing. The only thing out of her mouth would be, "Come and get these boys!" I could only reply, "I'm on my way." I would jump out of bed, wash my face, and brush my teeth. I needed to pick up the boys as soon as possible to appease Mother, knowing there would always be a next time. I usually made it to Mother's house in five minutes since she only lived 1.3 miles down the street. I measured the distance one day to see just how close together we lived. When I arrived, I thanked Mother profusely for allowing the boys to spend the night as she looked at me as if to say, "Yeah right!" Mother liked stuff so I typically brought along a gift or gave her some money as a token of our appreciation. Not because I had to but because it was the very least I could do.

Once when I picked the boys up, it was on a bright Saturday morning and Mother was in the middle of doing household chores. We chatted for a bit while the boys cleaned up after themselves. It looked like a tornado had spun around the basement and they had to put everything back in order before we were allowed to leave. It was either them or me and I was not about to pick up after them. They finally passed Mother's inspection of the basement and we were given the green light to leave.

Before I headed out the door and back to our house, I noticed a prescription bottle sitting on the coffee table. I casually asked Mother about it, and she explained that she had been started on a new medication for her arthritis. I didn't think much of it but told her it was important for her to keep track of what medications she was on. Mother liked to be in control and on top of things. She went on and on about how she knew her medications and how to take them and asked why was I was questioning her by asking "all these questions." Then she proceeded to tell me that she knew what was going on and that she could take care of herself.

I walked over to the coffee table and picked up the bottle of pills to read the prescription and said, "OK, Mother, what is the name of the new medication you're taking?" I sat the pills back down on the coffee table and gave Mother my full attention. When her response came to her, I could see the confidence on her face. She cocked her eyes at me and thought for a minute before blurting out, "I'm taking Viagra!" I thought I was hearing things. I paused to process what she'd said and realized I was not hearing things. My mouth fell wide open and a look of bewilderment blanketed my face that screamed "WTF!"

Mother must have seen my facial expression because she innocently asked, "What's wrong?" I said point blank, "Mother, you are *not* taking Viagra. The medication you are taking is Vioxx!" I paused to allow her to think about what she said. Mother looked at me and then at the pill bottle. When she realized her slip of the tongue or slip of the brain coupled with my response, we both looked at each other and broke out into hysterical laughter. It feels so good to stop everything you are doing and just laugh, and I'm glad we took the time. The days of laughter from Mother would grow fewer and farther between.

Chapter 5

I Remember ... *the Beauty Shop*

If you were looking for me and I was not at home or the gym, you could probably find me in the beauty shop where I had a standing appointment to get my hair styled by one of the best beautician in town, Dedra Adams. Although Dedra had a special talent when it came to cosmetology, she also had a propensity to be a bit unpredictable due to her lifestyle choices. It was nothing for her clients to show up for scheduled appointments only to find that Dedra was a no-show herself. Many of her clients remained loyal even when she became more unpredictable. There were many people praying and hoping for her release from the demons she struggled with. Dedra must have been in a good place in her life at the time because there I was waiting for her to work her magic on my hair. This hair of mine has always been short, thin and fragile so it was important for me to keep well coifed. Dedra was the best at doing this. The sense of liberation and confidence I felt after leaving the beauty shop made the financial and time sacrifices well worth it. I always left feeling better about myself no matter what was going on all around me. Having Dedra as a hair stylist was well worth the trips across town.

      This particular day that began as any other. I got up and piddled around the house. I was working twelve hour shifts and happened to be off. I was enjoying having the house to myself while Mike was at work and the boys were in school. I felt sleepy and decided to take a power nap before heading out to the beauty shop for a 3 o'clock hair appointment. I went ahead and got up and made it to the beauty shop with time to spare. I walked inside and took a seat. I said hello to everyone in the shop and started flicking through a hair style magazine to see if there was any styles I wanted to try. Noting seemed to interest me. Coming to the beauty shop was like going to a social club meeting. The clients and stylists were all acquainted with one another. Most of us either spent the time in the beauty shop reading, catching up on soap operas, gossiping or all of the above. There are unspoken rules in the beauty salon and they are:

1. The stylist knows when your appointment is.
2. Do not ask how long the stylist will be.
3. Do not give dirty looks to the stylist or that will prolong your wait time.
4. The stylist has the final say on any requested service.
5. What goes on in the beauty shop, stays in the beauty shop.
6. Stylists cannot work miracles.

The beauty shop was staffed with three stylists. At any given time, there would be anywhere from five to seven clients inside the shop with a couple of kids sprinkled in here and there. Each of us chatted about what had transpired in our lives since our last appointment. We also talked about what was going on in the community and in our personal lives. Everyone had kids, so there was always someone with a story to tell about what their children had or had not done. Each of us was in a relationship of some sort; some were looking for love, others were cohabitating or married. There always seemed to be something going on in somebody's life and we used the excessive amounts of time spent at the beauty shop to vent our frustrations or get opinions on whatever it was that was bothering us. Nine times out of ten, there was some knowledge to share or gain no matter where that information came from.

I was beginning to get antsy as I waited, but I dared not say anything. Typically, it takes approximately three hours for an appointment with Dedra, and the time varies based on the services required. A wash and set takes about two hours on a good day. A good day is when you arrive for your scheduled appointment with very little wait time for your name to be called. It also depended on what Dedra was already working on or how many heads were in front of you. A relaxer, cut, and color was at a minimum four-hour service time, so we learned to bring things along to keep us busy. I spent many hours catching up on paperwork while waiting for my turn at the beauty shop. This is time which I consider well spent.

Finally, Dedra called my name and began to work her magic on my hair. For some reason, when she washed my hair, she applied just enough pressure while scrubbing my scalp that made me relax and feel calm inside. The warm water trickling down to the nape of my neck made my hair straight and shiny. I sat in Dedra's chair and waited while she put the finishing touches on the client just ahead of me. Now, I had her full attention. It took Dedra only about ten minutes to roller-set my hair and I was under the hair dryer in a matter of minutes. I grabbed a *Jet* magazine to read while I sat underneath the dryer. I knew from experience that it would take approximately thirty minutes for my hair to thoroughly dry. I didn't have a care in the world.

Suddenly, my day was forever changed. I was jolted awake by my cellphone vibrating. I looked at the caller ID and saw the call was from

Mother. I helped myself out from under the dryer as my time was just about up anyway. I saw Dedra look at me out of the corner of my eye.

I answered my cellphone and said, "Hi, Ma." I was not prepared for what she said next: "I cannot find the church." I quizzically asked her what church she was talking about and she said, "We're supposed to sing tonight at Duncan Memorial."

It slowly came back to me. Mother and I were members of the same choir and we had an engagement to sing at Duncan Memorial Church on this particular Wednesday evening as guests for their fall revival celebration. I had no intention of participating. I could have attended, but I'd learned not to plan to do anything else when I had a hair appointment. I'm sure it boiled down to getting my hair done or singing in the choir.

By this time, Dedra had not yet called me up to finish up my hair, and I was not in any hurry since I needed to make sure Mother got to her destination. There I sat on my cellphone trying to explain to Mother the route to Duncan Memorial Church. I told her she needed to head toward town, to which she replied, "Which way is town?" I said, "What do you mean? Head towards Algonquin Parkway." "But I don't know where that is," Mother replied.

At this point, I am sure the look on my face was of complete astonishment as I stood up erect trying to fully process our conversation. I said, "Algonquin Parkway, the Big A Shopping Center— of course you know where that is." I felt my voice rising and my tone getting stern.

By this time, the expression on my face gave me away, and I noticed the beauty shop had become eerily quiet. It felt like I was in a bubble and all eyes were on me. I began to pace back and forth as my mind was racing. While still on the phone with Mother and trying to get her onto the right path, I methodically began to remove the rollers from my hair one at a time. This was a major stylist-client infraction—all but unheard of. No one said anything. With each roller removed, my mind searched for logic but none of this made any sense. In an instant, the once vibrant and bustling beauty shop was suddenly quiet as a cucumber as I continued my conversation with Mother. Everyone in the beauty shop could hear my side of the conversation, and I am sure they figured out pretty quickly that there was an issue.

"Do you think you can make it to Antioch" I asked Mother. "Yes, I see Antioch up the street," she said. "Well, wait for me at Antioch and I will be there in five minutes," I said as I got up and moved closer to Dedra's workstation. I gathered the rollers I had taken out of my hair and placed them in the bucket next to Dedra's workstation. I said, "I have got to go see about my mother" and abruptly left the beauty shop. Dedra only nodded for she and everyone else knew something must be going on. It takes a lot for a woman to leave the beauty shop with her hair not looking better than when she came in but my hair was the last thing on my mind. I was still trying to process our phone conversation. It was more than a bit troubling, to say the least.

All of this was a first for me. My hair was fresh out of the dryer, so my curls were considerably tight. I combed out my hair as much as I could as I drove to Antioch. It was almost 6:30 in the evening and the sun was just setting. A million things trampled through my mind on the seemingly interminable five-minute drive. When I pulled into the parking lot of Antioch, there sat Mother in her Volvo smiling widely. I pulled up next to her and instructed her to get into my car explaining that I would drive her to Duncan Memorial. As she got into the passenger seat, I was thinking, "What the hell is going on?"

As I drove Mother to Duncan Memorial, not only did my plans suddenly change, but so did our lives. It seemed the events of the last year or so was starting to add up and this is where we were. If it hadn't been clear to me before, it became abundantly clear that night that Mother had a problem much bigger than we could ever imagine.

I cannot recall what the preacher spoke about that night. I know there were people at Duncan Memorial that I spoke to, but I cannot for the life of me recall any details. I kept replaying the events of the day, as well as conversations and past occurrences that now made all of the sense in the world. That evening, Mother sang with the choir as she always did. I had never felt so alone while sitting in the middle of a room full of people fellowshipping before. I could do nothing except sit and stare blankly at nothing in particular. It was almost like an out-of-body experience.

All through the service, I kept a close eye on Mother. She didn't look any different and she really wasn't acting any different at that moment. She looked like her old self, like the mother I was accustomed to seeing. But I knew very well that something was both different and just plain wrong. No one at the church that evening had a clue of the turmoil that was going on inside of me. Mother was now in the house of the Lord and I thought there was no better place for both of us to be. We both needed more help than we ever had needed before.

Church is where I could find peace in the midst of a storm. The storm that was brewing inside me was overpowering my ability to concentrate on anything. I tried to focus on God but my Mother and her behavior that day had my stomach tied in knots.

I willed myself not think about how bad I thought things were and how afraid I was. Suddenly, there was a sense of calmness that came over me. Mother and I were where we were supposed to be. At the end of the service, I drove Mother back to Antioch to pick up her car. We didn't say much on the drive back. As we passed Algonquin Parkway, I couldn't help but say, "See, there's Algonquin Parkway. Do you remember Algonquin Parkway?" "Yes," she said, laughing a little. To this day, I am not sure if Mother knew what she was laughing at but I could not find any humor in any of the events of the past couple of hours. I was numb.

When we finally arrived back at Antioch, I told Mother that I would follow her home to which she replied, "You don't have to do that." I said, "I know I don't, but I want to." In typical Mother fashion, she said, "Well, if you must." We lived so close to one another that it only made sense for me to follow Mother to make sure she got home safely. I watched as she pulled into her driveway. I didn't continue on to my house until I saw that she was safely inside her door. I drove home feeling totally exhausted from the events of the day. I was at a complete loss and didn't know what to do or say. I simply didn't want to be bothered with anyone or anything. I went straight up to my bedroom and ran some warm bath water. Thank God the boys were in the basement and Mike was on the couch watching television. I made myself a cocktail, got into bed and fell asleep.

We all had come a long way from the projects, and this should have been the time for Mother to enjoy the fruits of her labor. Our family has been blessed with good genes and physical health. However, there have long been rumblings about family members "losing their mind," but that's one of the topics we didn't talk about.

Chapter 6

I Remember ... *the Evaluation*

You would have thought that it was Black Friday all over again. It was a cold, overcast, and gloomy morning that seemed to mimic our feelings. This was the day that my siblings and I cleared our schedules and made it a point to accompany Mother to her doctor's appointment. Everyone knew what the outcome would be but for some reason we felt the need to hear if from an outside source. Perhaps we needed to get a professional opinion so that each of us could hear with our own ears and not someone's interpretation. But mostly, we all really only wanted to make sure that Mother would be OK. The moment of truth was finally here.

Of course, it was a doctor's office, so we expected to wait. I arrived first and sat quietly by myself in the waiting room. I found a nice quiet corner and meditated for a few minutes. I had left work in the middle of the morning and had to rush to make it on time so I needed a few minutes to relax. Knowing that our family is habitually late for everything, I waited patiently for Felicia to arrive with Mother. Although I had several minutes to prepare myself for this moment, I still wasn't quite sure what to expect. When our family gathers for a discussion, anything can happen and it usually does. It would not be the first time that I was embarrassed by something one of my siblings said or did. Lord knows, I'm sure they could say the exact same thing about me. Mike says we get it honest, because we act just like Mother which is mostly a good thing. But, there are times when due to Mother's behavior, I felt inclined to apologize in advance for what she might say or do.

By the loud noises in the hallway, I guessed someone in our family had arrived. I looked up when the office door was pulled open and in walked

Felicia and Mother. Mother looked exceptionally well. Her hair and makeup were perfect. If Mother asked you how she looked and you responded "OK" or "alright" she would re-do something to obtain the response she had been looking for in the first place, which was that she looked fabulous, amazing or incredible.

    Mother and Felicia sat across from me and we all waited without saying much. Vance and Shonie came in next and joined us in the waiting room. Charlene was the last to arrive and came straight there from her night-shift job. We all sat and waited for Mother's name to be called. There was small talk between us as we tried to stay calm and relaxed. We made it a point to talk in our soft voices as the waiting room grew louder and louder with each passing moment. It must've been our nervous energy that got everyone talkative and excited. We had to remind one another that we were in a doctor's office with sick people. We finally stopped talking altogether and thumbed through some of the magazines scattered here and there to pass the time.

    After about ten minutes, the medical assistant swung open the door and called out Mother's name. I'm sure they called on us so quickly because they wanted to clear the waiting room of so many extraneous people. We all marched in one after the other with Mother nestled in the middle of us. It reminded me of when we were children and Mother had us trained in how to walk, how to talk, what to say and when to say it. It makes sense for family members to accompany an elderly parent to the doctor but Mother had all of her children with her.

We each felt the need to hear and see for ourselves what the doctor said and did. We had lost the ability to trust in one another. I was beginning to see many things that were once held in high esteem in the family disintegrate to levels of insignificance that not only puzzled but troubled me. I couldn't put my finger on it, but I could tell that we were in for a rude awakening.

Each of us took a place in the small exam room which seemed to shrink by the minute. I stood because there was no room to sit. Felicia sat in a chair. Mother sat on the exam table mostly listening and occasionally laughing at Vance's jokes. Charlene said she didn't mind standing and thought it would keep her more alert. Vance found a place to sit on a stool and Shonie sort of paced in a small circle. No one asked her to sit down; we knew she needed this outlet to calm herself. Even though Shonie's pacing was making me more nervous than I already was, I made it a point not to comment for fear of causing more stress and uneasiness. I probably would not have minded so much if the room wasn't so small.

Mother had been a patient in this practice for about thirty years. Her longtime primary care doctor, Dr. Phillip Feitels, had been taking care of her during that whole time. When he entered the exam room, I don't think he had been warned that the entire family was with Mother. He had a surprised look on his face and seemed impressed that we could fit so many people in an exam room. There was barely enough room for each of us so we made sure Dr. Feitels had enough space to examine and evaluate Mother. He graciously acknowledged everyone in the room. After brief introductions and pleasantries, the doctor turned his attention to

Mother. Dr. Feitels was a well-respected physician in the community and, since Mother was in such good health, she would only see him on rare occasions for check-ups and a few ailments here and there. If she trusted him after all of those years, we felt we could trust and respect his opinion and assessment of this situation in which we found ourselves.

    As Dr. Feitels began the evaluation, he first asked Mother if it was alright to have "all these people" in the room while he did his examination. Mother replied, "Of course, these are my children." She laughed and so did we. Dr. Feitels then asked Mother if she knew why we were all here with her today and she said, "They're concerned about me and they've been talking about me." He asked, "What have they been saying?" Mother was evasive as ever and said, "Y'all tell him."

    Felicia began. "You see, stuff has been happening to Mama," she said, and then she began to cry. Between sobs, she explained how Mother had been having trouble with her memory and gave specific instances of her forgetfulness. Felicia sobbed harder when she explained how Mother recently slipped and fell while in the shower. It was extremely difficult to hear the gory details, some of which we all were not aware of. Felicia had an insight to everything that was going on since she and Mother shared a home. As she talked, it brought into perspective how each of us had been in various stages of denial about the actual state of Mother's health. Mother sat quietly while we did most of the talking about various things we had observed. She listened to everything that was being said; I think she had been worried about herself as well.

As Dr. Feitels began with his evaluation, everyone started jumping in and answering his questions that were intended for Mother. Felicia was the main culprit. When Dr. Feitels tested Mother's cognition by asking her what day it was, Felicia replied, "Friday." Vance said, "I didn't even know what day it is," and we all had a good laugh that seemed to lighten the intensity in the air. We definitely needed a reason to laugh. When it happened again, I finally had to remind everyone that the questions were for Mother and to let the doctor do his job. "I know, I know," was the reply, along with everyone nodding in agreement.

If Dr. Feitels thought this appointment was going to be short and easy, he soon realized it was quite the opposite. He tried again: "Who is the president?" Mother shot back: "Barack Obama!" He then gave Mother a series of words and asked her to remember them until later. Next, he handed her a clipboard with a piece of paper and a pencil and asked her to draw a picture of a clock. It seemed easy enough, but boy were we shocked. This is where Mother really struggled. It was as if she did not know where to begin or how to accomplish this task. It was difficult to watch her looking lost and not able to figure out where to begin, let alone finish. I'm certain it didn't help with all of us in the background saying, "Ma, you know how to do this." Then someone else said, "Be quiet, and let her do it herself." Then there was a moment of silence as we all watched Mother scribble illegible marks on the paper.

As Dr. Feitels continued his examination, each of us had the opportunity to see what Mother drew. The depiction of a clock was heartbreaking; our hearts sank one at a time as we each saw firsthand the true state of the situation. This was the "wow" moment for all of us. We were stunned, and nobody said anything throughout the remainder of the evaluation. We cheered the tests she passed and sulked when she was not successful. Sadly, there was mostly sulking and frankly not much to cheer for. Mother had to have known that her every move was being measured by everyone in the room with the utmost scrutiny. I cannot imagine what she must've felt.

    Dr. Feitels did a few more tests but I think we had pretty much seen enough. During the examination, it was also noted that Mother had lost about fifteen pounds since her last doctor's visit just three months before. And Mother didn't need to lose any weight. In fact, her jeans were beginning to sag on her. Dr. Feitels asked Mother if she was eating and if she remembered to eat. We did not know for sure if Mother even ate lunch during the day. At this particular point, Felicia was still working so she and Mother would have breakfast and dinner together, but not lunch. We knew for certain that Mother was losing weight rapidly and we could only figure that she was not eating as she should.

    Dr. Feitels finally asked Mother if she could recall the series of words he had asked her to remember earlier. Mother searched and searched her mind but couldn't find the words she was looking for. I think at this point it was painfully clear to us that Mother was in worse shape than we initially feared. She finally said she didn't remember the words, and we told her that it was OK. Dr. Feitels didn't have to say anything more, but I am so glad he did because we all needed to hear it. He confirmed what we each suspected: that Mother had Alzheimer's disease. There, it was out for the whole family to hear. My nursing experience hadn't prepared me to be on this side of a terrible diagnosis.

Everyone was eerily quiet while Dr. Feitels explained the disease and treatment options. Next, he adjusted some of Mother's current medications and started her on some new pills that could help slow the progression of Alzheimer's. He stepped out of the exam room to retrieve some samples for Mother. We all agreed to try the medication; after all, this was the only practical option since there is no cure for Alzheimer's.

Even though we kind of knew what to expect, the diagnosis was an absolute kick in the gut to each of us. We were dumbfounded, but at least we could go about fighting this thing called Alzheimer's and getting Mother the treatment she needed. We sat in silence in the exam room for a few minutes trying to absorb everything we had heard, seen and felt. After what seemed like a long time but was really only about five minutes, Dr. Feitels brought in the new prescriptions and samples. We collected our belongings and proceeded to leave. We thanked the doctor for his patience with us and for his care of Mother. It was a long, slow procession from the exam room back out to the waiting room, where Felicia made sure Mother got properly checked out. The waiting room atmosphere was significantly different from when we first arrived. Saddled with a new diagnosis for Mother, along with many thoughts racing through our heads, nobody said anything. You could've heard a pin drop. I think we were all numb. I cannot imagine what Mother must've been feeling or thinking.

Felicia and Mother left together to get her prescriptions filled. Vance and Shonie followed soon after with their heads bowed low. They didn't say much except a quick good-bye. As I drove out of the parking garage and tried to absorb everything, I found myself recalling how much of Mother's recent behaviors and actions now made sense. I went back to work and tried to concentrate.

Felicia called a couple hours later to say she had gotten the prescriptions filled and had started Mother on her new medications. Well, good, I thought, hoping that the medications would buy us some valuable and precious time. I never dreamed how close and personal I would become with this awful disease.

Chapter 7

I Remember ... *the Restaurant*

It had been a particularly rough day at work, and I came home to an even rougher patch in our marriage. Mike and I were struggling, to say the least. We had each brought two sons into our marriage—we had no children together—and there were many times when our family was split down the middle: his and hers. And, we were struggling with our finances. No matter how easy or how amicable life should have been for me and Mike, everything seemed to be a struggle. We lost sight of us and couldn't figure out how to get back to being us. He didn't nudge and neither did I, so the struggle was real.

No matter how difficult things got in our marriage, Mike and I were of one accord when we felt we needed to get out of the house and forget about everything. In spite of the arguments and insults, we managed to put all of that aside and enjoy ourselves every once in a while.

Our favorite indulgence and one thing we could agree on was happy hour. If two people needed an hour or two for some happy, it was us. This was our opportunity to get away from the house, away from the kids, and away from our problems, and drown ourselves in some good Mexican food and cheap margaritas. El Nopalito was a neighborhood restaurant where we could get our fix for both. The food was delicious, and the margaritas were tasty. We like our margaritas on the rocks and with salt. If Mike and I couldn't agree on anything else, this was one of the few things that we didn't feel the need to argue about.

We jumped at the opportunity to get out of the house. Maybe it was because this was our escape from reality, if only for a couple of hours. This date was worth the money we shouldn't have been spending due to the fact that we had more than enough bills piling up in our junk drawer. But on this particular day, it was all about us.

For far too long, everything had been about the kids. Luckily, the boys, as we affectionately called them, got along great, as you would expect boys to do. They ranged in ages from ten to seventeen and they drove us absolutely crazy at times. But overall they were pretty good kids. Of course, since there were four boys in our family, we could expect to find even more boys from the neighborhood crammed in our basement on any given day. If they were not having a party in the basement, they were having a brawl. It sort of scared me thinking about what could be going on in the basement, and I dared not venture downstairs. I didn't want to know what they were doing, but I knew they were always up to something. However, there was also a peace of mind in knowing that the boys were at least safely tucked away downstairs even if they probably were up to no good. I know, it is supposed to be all about the kids. The way I look at it, the boys had it made. After all, they had a nice home, a kitchen full of food, fairly nice clothes, parents who loved them, and the privilege to have choices and to make choices. Heck, when I was young, it was Mother's way or the highway. Kids today just don't get it.

Mike and I arrived at El Nopalito at about 5 o'clock in the afternoon, just in time to partake in the two-for-one happy hour. Everyone deserves a little happiness once in a while; this was our opportunity and we took full advantage of it. We decided to sit inside the restaurant instead of outside on the covered patio. We sat at a table right in the middle of the restaurant. Our waitress was a cute, young lady who appeared to be of Mexican descent based on her appearance and her accent. She was extremely pretty and pleasant. She asked Mike and me what we wanted to drink. When I asked what the special was, she said, "We have two-for-one margaritas." That was music to my ears, and we both ordered margaritas. I assumed that the waitress would bring us each one margarita, but to my delight she brought us out two margaritas apiece. My eyes lit up as we drank the margaritas, licked the salt, and snacked on the chips and salsa. This was the first time in a long while that Mike and I had the opportunity to have a civil conversation with one another. If only for this moment, we were the happiest couple in town. Life was good for the moment.

After we ate more chips and salsa than we probably should have, we ordered our dinners. Mike opted for the fajitas; I ordered the fish tacos. Both meals came with the standard side dishes of refried beans and Spanish rice. We also felt inclined to order another round of margaritas for both of us. By the time our food came, we were primed and ready to eat some food to soak up some of the tequila we had been drinking. We both were only able to eat about half of our meals; when you fill up on margaritas, chips, and salsa, there's not much room for anything else.

After talking for an hour of more, we decided it was time to head back home. We motioned for our waitress to ask for our check and some to-go boxes. While waiting for our waitress to return, Mike and I continued to talk and someway, somehow, the discussion turned to Mother. Out of nowhere and before I could do anything, I suddenly burst out in tears. I tried to suppress the feeling that came over me, but I couldn't. It was as if the magnitude of everything I had been suppressing for so long was much bigger and much stronger than I could withstand. The tequila probably made me a bit more relaxed and more vulnerable than I suspected.

My crying episode was not subtle at all but a full-fledged, gut-wrenching cry, where my face was distorted and my tears seemingly flowed with ease. Mike asked what was wrong, and I said "Ma has Alzheimer's, and it's so unfair." Just saying the words caused me to cry even more. Now, other people were beginning to notice. Mike appeared to be stunned as I sat crying in the middle of the restaurant. He didn't know what to do, so he just sat and just stared at me. (Mike tends to clam up when things get tense, and I'd learned to accept him just being there.) I tried to gather myself but the tears just kept coming. There was nothing I could do to suppress this overwhelming feeling; I had to get it out of my system. The harder I tried to hold back my sobs, the more they came. Now, more people in the restaurant were staring at us. We must've been a sight with me crying like a baby and Mike staring blankly across the table from me.

When our waitress returned, her gaze was focused on me. She said, in a calm and soothing voice, "Señora, what is the matter?" while looking at Mike as if he was the culprit. I quickly said, "I'm OK. I'm just sad because my mother...." I stopped because I couldn't say it. I didn't want to give in to it. I definitely didn't want to believe it. But then I blurted out, "My mother has Alzheimer's."

The waitress stared at me and then looked at Mike while comforting me by caressing my shoulder. She asked if she could do anything to make me feel better. I thanked her for her kindness and told her there was nothing she or anybody could do. I assured her that I would be OK, and she told me to let her know if I needed anything at all. After a few minutes, I regained my composure and finished my margarita. Mike paid our bill, and I made it a point to again thank our waitress for being so caring and attentive. It made me feel good that a stranger actually took the time to show she cared. I know I couldn't repay her kindness, but I made sure she had a good tip to show just how much I appreciated her.

Maybe that was what my spirit needed. A little kindness and attention can go a long way. Mike and I left the restaurant to head back home. It was a quiet drive to our house, back to our boys, back to our lives, and back to reality. I must say that I did feel a bit refreshed after my crying episode. The margaritas probably helped a little, too.

Every once in a while, my emotions will get the best of me, and my only recourse is to cry. And sometimes, it is more of a sob. I tend to refrain from allowing people to see me cry. Most people think I'm a tough and strong person, which I can agree with.

But I also get weak sometimes. When those moments come, I find comfort while crying in the shower. It is such a refreshing release. The sound of the clear water jetting out of the showerhead and beating against the tile floor drowns out my sobs. The constant flow of water streaming from the faucet onto my face obliterates the tears as they cascade freely from eyes. The watered-down tears then flow down the drain as if they never existed. I give myself just enough time to have a good cry, which is about as long as a five-minute shower.

During this time, I make it a point to get out all of my frustrations out and have a pity party with myself. By the time my shower is complete, I use my towel to dry myself off and especially to dry away all my tears. This ritual recharges and sustains me until the next time I feel the need to have just one more cry.

Chapter 8

I Remember ... *the Light*

Mother was cruising along nicely and right about 70 years old when the thief decided to become more aggressive. As Mother's disease progressed, the impact on her, my siblings, and me was evident to everyone. We would never be the same. The drastic psychological and perplexing physical changes that we saw happening to Mother were far too much for any of us to bear. Unfortunately, we didn't handle the challenges of life well. We did a terrible job of managing our familial relationships and responsibilities.

Because I'm a nurse, I was tasked with much of Mother's care and with ensuring that her health condition was being treated appropriately. My siblings asked for my opinion anytime Mother's medication regimen changed or if there was a noticeable decline in her cognition. I offered my professional opinion to the best of my abilities. It would've been nice if they listened more and talked less. I didn't think they realized just how bad things were about to become. I tried to prepare them for how ugly things were going to get, but they weren't hearing me. I finally got tired of fighting a losing battle. I figured it was best if I kept my mouth closed and did as I was told for the most part.

Health challenges are extremely difficult to first accept and then process, especially when the crisis impacts your loved one. I came to learn that if the foundation is not solid, and I do mean solid, the cracks and stressors of a crisis will soon collapse everything that was once believed to be functional and unbreakable. I was almost dumbfounded by some of the things that were said, done, or implied. Our family dynamics changed in a way that I didn't see coming. There comes a point where you clearly see the various components of people you've known all of your life only to find that everyone has an agenda. When facts finally protruded through the shield of conflict, many things became abundantly clear. It took a lot of time, tears, and turmoil to realize that it was never about any of us in the first place. It should've always been about what was best for Mother.

Communication had never been a strong trait in our family. Although we tend to talk loud and with a lot of passion, I think it is a way for us to fit in and be heard. For the most part, we either had no communication, poor communication, or total miscommunication.

I should've known immediately that something was up when I received the group text from Felicia requesting a family meeting regarding Mother. I didn't know what to expect. We had never had a family meeting before, so I knew something was brewing. I remember thinking that Shonie and Felicia must be up to something again, but I couldn't put my finger on what this meeting could be about.

On the day of the family meeting, everyone except Vance arrived at the house that Mother and Felicia shared. We waited for Vance to arrive as long as possible by filling the time with small talk and actually enjoying one another's company. Mother sat quietly on the couch and was agreeable when addressed. I think she knew that something serious was about to happen. It became evident that Vance wasn't going to make it, so we proceeded with the meeting without him. Shonie started first like she was in charge—as she always did. She cut straight to the point and pretty much said that it was time that we all needed to take an active part in Mother's care. Shonie did most of the talking, but it was obvious that she and Felicia had been discussing exactly what they wanted to see happen. Everyone listened. We all knew that she was right. We had assumed that Mother was doing just fine. Little did we know that Mother's dependence on Felicia had escalated to the point where Felicia not only needed a break but deserved a break.

Shonie explained that Felicia was wearing herself out physically and mentally trying to care for Mother. Well, of course, she needed help. I had tried to tell them a couple of years before about care options. My suggestion to look into adult day care for Mother had been shot down, no questions asked. In fact, they didn't want to hear of it, so I dropped the subject. Many times I had seen the effects of caregiver burnout and warned our family that it could happen to anyone.

Felicia had subsequently retired from her job so that she had more time to devote to caring for Mother. At the time, we thought this was a blessing. We all lived with blinders on because I think we were hoping things were better than we feared. The toll of living with and caring for Mother twenty-four hours a day, day in and day out, had become too much. We should've realized this sooner and provided more support for Felicia and for Mother.

Of course, we all agreed to do our part to help with Mother's care. Everyone agreed that Felicia would continue to care for Mother during the week. We developed a schedule where on weekends we would take turns caring for Mother in our own homes. We excluded Felicia from the weekend rotation since she had the bulk of the responsibility during the week. The schedule was such that on your assigned weekend, you were to pick up Mother on Friday by 5 o'clock in the afternoon and drop her back at her home on Sunday evening. That sounded fair enough. It all made perfect sense and was the very least we could do, I suppose. We made a schedule and informed Vance of the plan and his place in the weekend rotation. As everyone left the meeting, we were all in agreement for once. I was glad the meeting went well. I'm sure Mother was proud of how we handled ourselves, even though she didn't say much.

    I went back to my house and thought about the events of the day. I was torn by our new plan for Mother's care. It was long overdue, but it would be an adjustment for all of us. I wasn't particular fond of the idea of Mother being passed around every weekend, but what other choice did we have? I learned to get over that pretty quickly. I had to adjust my life a bit. I made it a point to clearly mark on my calendar the designated weekends I was to care for Mother. It was weird for a while, but my family and friends understood that my responsibilities were changing and I had to do things a bit differently. While my friends had commitments to their children and grandchildren, my commitment was to my mother. When I was asked to go somewhere or do something on the weekends that I had Mother, my reply was, "I have my mom this weekend." No questions were asked, because they got it.

    We had implemented the new care schedule and things were going well. You could see the change in Felicia as she had some time for herself for the first time in a long time. Things were much better for everyone in the family. As I jumped out of bed to go to church one Sunday morning, I had some pep in my step. This was my weekend without Mother, and I felt I could do anything I wanted. So,

I went to church and enjoyed the sermon that day. Everyone asked how Mother was doing, and I replied that she was doing OK.

When I left church, it had begun to rain. I dreaded it, but I had to stop at the drugstore for a few items. I pulled into the parking lot and as I hurried out of the car, I thought I heard a voice calling my name. I couldn't be sure because I was parked along a busy street. All of a sudden, I heard it again. Someone was calling for me. I couldn't imagine who on earth it could be; at the time, Mike and I were staying on a side of town where none of our friends or family frequented. Still, the voice sounded vaguely familiar, and the twang in the voice revealed that this was none other than my sister-in-law, Claire, Vance's wife. What in the world was she doing on this side of town? I stopped in my tracks, turned around, and hurried over to her car as she was just about to drive off.

It turned out that Mother was in the backseat. She had seen me heading into the drugstore and said, "That's my daughter." Claire said she had no idea what Mother was talking about, but then she looked up and saw me walking. "She said it, didn't she?" Claire asked the other occupants in the car. They all confirmed the story.

As I stepped closer and peered inside the back seat of the car, I saw Mother snuggly wrapped in an oversized coat next to a couple other people. Apparently, they had decided to make a pit stop at the drugstore on their way home from their church. This was Vance and Claire's weekend to take care of Mother.

I thought Mother looked gray. Her hair was gray, her coat was gray, her eyes were gray, and the sky was gray. It was another gray moment in a gray kind-of day. I was glad that I didn't see Mother at our church earlier because, her appearance was not up to church standards, as far as I was concerned. To me, Mother looked like a little old lady with Alzheimer's, and it hurt to see her like this. I never expected to ever see Mother look like she did then.

Mother had very high standards of dress and appearance, and this was not anywhere near her standards. If she could say or do anything about how she looked, things would be very different. While growing up, if I'd wanted to go out looking like she did now, she would've said, "You're not going with me looking like that," at which point I would immediately have run inside to change into something acceptable to be seen in public. The way Mother looked then, I would've stayed at home myself, but it wasn't my weekend to make that call.

Although Claire repeated that Mother said, "That's my daughter," the only thing I could get out of her was "Fine" when I asked her how she was doing. For Mother to call me by name at this point, which had not happened in a very long time, would've been very surprising. Oh how I would have loved to hear Mother call my name just one more time. I came to the realization that the thief robs us all of something, whether we have the disease or live with a loved one who has it. The thief has a way of not only screwing up the affected person's head, but also testing the family that is left to continue on with life despite the disease's toll on the mind, body, spirit and faith.

To me, Mother's inability to say my name was one of the most heartbreaking milestones we passed. I would ask her to tell me my name, and she would say, "I don't know," which was her easy way out of situations. This was puzzling to me because I wondered how she knew that she didn't know. I mean, "I don't know" is an appropriate response, and she knew enough to know that she didn't know. But this disease will have you questioning everything and none of it will make any sense.

Little did I know then that what I was doing was the absolute worst thing I could've asked of Mother. Sometimes, what we want to see and feel from our loved ones gets in the way of what is best for them in their fragile state. I know I shouldn't have been questioning or testing Mother, but I couldn't help it. I yearned for her to remember my name.

I gradually learned to accept that the opportunity to hear Mother call me by my given name had been long gone. Over time, she simply said my name less and less until she didn't say it anymore. Even though I truly think Mother did know my name, it was easier for her to say she didn't know it because she just couldn't get the words out.

Mother was still Mother no matter what. Everyone who has a mother wants their mother to know who they are, recognize them, and call them by name.

When people ask the stupid questions like "Does she know who you are?" I have to take a deep breath before responding. This is a difficult question to answer and to explain. My fear is that we are becoming more and more culturally insensitive, which is scary. My reply to this rather tacky question is a resounding "Yes!" I try to make them aware that Mother is not able to call me by name, but she knows who I am. I go on to explain that my name gets trapped in her head but that she is well aware that I am her daughter. I then delve into the broken synapses in Mother's brain and compare them to our broken hearts, and people usually get it. Only Mother's brokenness cannot be mended. Not only can we not help her, but she cannot help herself.

A part of me would like to think that Mother is lucky not to realize the hand she has been dealt. The other part of me fears that Mother knows very well the dilemma she is in but has no way out of. It's ironic that we very much want our loved ones to remember us but we don't want them to be aware of their cognitive decline. It's only natural that we would want the best for everyone.

There in front of the drugstore, I chatted with Claire and Mother and the other occupants in the car for a few minutes. They all had questions about Mother and why she did the things she did and what could we do to curtail her behaviors. I so hated where this conversation was going.

Everyone had noticed certain behavioral changes in Mother. How could you not notice when someone does things in front of you that are simply appalling? Your natural reaction is to be filled with disgust, even anger, at the absolute lack of self-control. It matters not who should happen to see one of these awkward behaviors. When people looked in shock at an ill-advised behavior, I would simply reply, "She has Alzheimer's" and keep the conversation moving. Most people usually get it. These people understand immediately and look the other way. Others are so intrigued that they stare to see what this Alzheimer's stuff is all about.

I'm sure they soon find out that Alzheimer's is an awful, ugly disease that cuts at the core of the individual and gradually robs them of themselves. This thief is ruthless. I was absolutely mortified when Mother picked her nose or ate with her fingers in public. It got to the point where I stopped asking Mother to stop the behavior because she couldn't remember what it was she did in the first place. How funny is that? So many people spend so much time trying to get people with Alzheimer's to do or stop doing something, but the person with the disease doesn't even realize what it was they did in the first place. It's a losing battle and a humbling reality

      Personally, I'd rather take a bullet to the head or have cancer than be cursed with Alzheimer's. Everyone seems to know what cancer is. There is a push for people to walk, race, ride a bike, and feel compassion for those impacted by cancer—and they should. With Alzheimer's, on the other hand, people tend to want to think it doesn't exist or that it'll somehow just go away if we ignore it. I'm thrilled to know that people can be cured of some diseases. For Alzheimer's, there is no cure—yet! A person diagnosed with Alzheimer's gradually diminishes in cognition and self until they finally die. I sometimes pray that Mother will be taken out of her misery. I know she is miserable, as anyone in this state must be. There comes a time when we must acknowledge what is best not for us, but for the person living with Alzheimer's.

      Before I let Claire and Mother continue on their way, I couldn't resist the urge to ask Mother if she knew my name. Her reply, "I don't know," devastated me again. It was as if my heart was left broken yet again.

Chapter 9

I Remember ... *the Church*

Our family had been active members at Antioch Baptist Church for over thirty years. Mike was the director of the men's choir, I served as the church clerk, Vance was a deacon, and Mother was a member of both the mass choir and the liturgical dance ministry before Alzheimer's came roaring into our lives. Antioch was small and intimate, and everyone either knew you or was related to you. Many of the families had a deep history with the church that go back for several generations. Our family was welcomed as members with open arms, and we soon found ourselves with a church family that was more like an extension of our own family. It was actually one of Shonie's friends who invited us to Antioch to visit. We liked it so much that the entire family ended up joining. We did what Christians do: We went to church. We supported our pastor and his teachings. We paid our tithes and went home and did it all over again the next week. This routine seemed to work for a while.

     Before Mother got Alzheimer's, she loved being involved in church activities. If being the president of the mass choir wasn't enough, Mother felt the need to express herself by performing dramatizations of poems by Maya Angelou for special church programs. She would immerse herself into character and the message of the poems. Her performances left you mesmerized. Initially, during these performances, Mother commanded the stage with her presence, her costume, her makeup, and her voice. Her ability to use her tone and reenactment of a poem made you think that Mother was telling the poem just as Maya Angelou intended for the interpretation. The congregation heaped praise onto Mother in appreciation for her dramatic skills. The stage was a place that Mother excelled. It was as if she were free to express herself and show a different side of herself. It was obvious that Mother loved the stage and the stage loved her. As Mother recited poems, she used her hands and her body to bring it to life. She had no problem keeping the audience engaged while at the same time delivering a powerful message.

    I remember one of her last performances. I was strategically seated on a pew in close proximity to Mother in an effort to feed her the words to the poem when the words wouldn't come to her. I didn't think anything of it because some of these poems were extremely long and Mother was able to memorize most of them. On this particular day, Mother was cruising along nicely and she got stumped. Unfortunately, as she was moving around the sanctuary, she had managed to move so far away from me and couldn't hear me as I tried to help her find her place.

    There was a spotlight shining brightly on Mother; everywhere she went, the spotlight followed her. I noticed that the spotlight was shining directly in her face while she was trying to recite her poem. Mother began to fumble over her words. Just when I thought she was going to fall apart, she had a ram-in-the-bush moment. In the blink of an eye and in full character, Mother attributed her lapse to the spotlight. She did this in such a manner that was so like her that everyone in the audience broke out into laughter. I could only shake my head in amazement at how she could turn things around and make them work out in her favor.

    Well, it didn't take long for Mother's forgetfulness to be noticed by other members in the church. It was shortly after this that "they" realized Mother had something going on with her memory.

"They" were the people outside of our immediate family.

For some reason, Mother didn't want anyone to know she had Alzheimer's, not even her siblings. People can be so unforgiving, especially when they don't have all the necessary information to make an informed decision. Mother was still the president of the mass choir when things started going downhill fast. Unfortunately, she wasn't able to carry out some of the duties this role required. I had to explain over and over again to choir members that there were some things that Mother couldn't do, such as coordinate the Wednesday night potluck. It simply was not going to happen if they were relying on Mother. I wanted to scream, "Do you not get it?" I now know that they truly didn't get it at all.

Once, I calmly explained to the members of the choir that Mother was able to participate in activities but would not be able to coordinate the details of an event. Just when I was about to get my point across, Mother chimed in and said that I couldn't tell her what she could and could not do. I sat down in exasperation. I didn't respond and only shook my head. Everyone just looked at me as if I was speaking a foreign language.

It almost broke my heart when Sister Toby came to me and said, "Your mother couldn't find her purse, and then she got agitated and very upset." I thanked Sister Toby and told her that Mother had Alzheimer's and that we would take care of her. The secret was out.

It was a very sad day when Mother had to give up being a part of the liturgical dance ministry. Not many 67-year-olds take up liturgical dancing, but of course Mother did. She did a fantastic job in this ministry while she could. I remember her waving her flag during the dance routines with such vigor and passion that I swear a few people actually ducked their heads as Mother gracefully sauntered past them. Heck, I even ducked a few times myself. If those poor people hadn't gotten out of the way, I'm afraid of what may have happened. Of course, Mother was totally oblivious to any of this. I wish you could've seen the look on my face as I watched Mother roar through the sanctuary like a fiery cat. With each completed performance, I breathed a sigh of relief and praised God there were no casualties.

When Mother realized she would have to give up the dance ministry, she said, "Y'all are leaving me out." I tried to explain that it was time. She didn't understand my rationale, and I really couldn't explain it well enough to assuage her disappointment.

One of the most difficult interactions I have ever witnessed was after church one Sunday afternoon. One of Mother's longtime friends was particularly chatty with her. I was feeling a little over-protective. Mother found comfort in having one of us with her. I think she knew that something was going on but she couldn't put her finger on it. We tended to stick closely by Mother mostly to help her out of awkward situations and to look out for her best interests. Frankly, I found that most people simply didn't understand what Alzheimer's was in the first place and were trying to better understand what was happening to Mother.

As we were leaving church, everyone gathered in the vestibule to chat. Well, Sandy made a beeline over to Mother, who was always within an arm's reach of me. Sandy said hello to me and to

Mother. And then, before I could interject, she proceeded to ask Mother when her birthday was.

It wasn't an innocent question at all. I knew exactly where she was going. I was completely caught off guard and for a moment I was speechless. Mother still had some fight in her and spat back, "I don't know when my birthday is." I was finally able to gather my words and say, "Her birthday is in August. It's the twenty third." "That's right," Mother said. I took Mother by the hand and we marched outside to leave for home. My blood was boiling as I helped her into the car and we started for home. I was furious that Sandy had the nerve to test Mother like that. And that's exactly what it was: a test.

How dare she and why would she? It took me a few days to calm down. I came to realize that Sandy didn't understand that asking a person with Alzheimer's a question is the absolute worst thing a person can do. I liken it to asking a person with lung disease if they would like to catch their breath a person with some other challenging illness if they would like to be whole or normal. It took me a long time to get over this. The fact is, this occurred and is attributed to pure and unadulterated ignorance. The Bible says we have to be better so I tried. I had to put on the full spiritual armor to get my mind and my heart right. I wanted to say something to Sandy, but I am glad I didn't because it certainly would've come out the wrong way.

I soon found myself doing a lot of questioning. I couldn't help but to question why and how Alzheimer's happened to Mother of all of the people in the whole wide world. Why Mother? Why not Mother?

Mother continued to go to church every day she felt up to it. There were good days, and there were some not so good days. At this stage of the disease, getting Mother to church was a major chore. When I did garner the energy and the time to take her to church, I had to start my day extra early to get her fed, dressed, and ready. Then, I had to get myself ready. Caring for Mother was more strenuous and taxing than taking care for a baby. At least an infant is smaller in stature and when there is a struggle, you have the upper hand. When people who have Alzheimer's get set in their way, you may as well give up because they will fight you and they will win.

I gradually learned to let things go. It was a tough lesson but a good lesson. You see, when Mother made up her mind about something, this had a significant impact on what we were or were not going to do. I had to realize that the battle between us was really between me and Alzheimer's. I had to plan accordingly and be prepared to submit. If you're like me and hate losing to anyone or anything, Alzheimer's can be very humbling. No one wins with this disease—never has, never will.

By the time we finally made it to church, I would be completely worn out. I made a special effort to take Mother to church as much as I possibly could. She enjoyed being at church, in the house of the Lord. There were many days that when we finally pulled into the church parking lot, my thoughts immediately shifted to, now if we could just get her out of the car it would make all of the time and effort worth it.

It wasn't long thereafter that Mother had to relinquish her treasured role as president of the mass choir. For the first time in her life, she needed us like she never needed us before. I can hear her very clearly in my head: "You think I depend on you?" I only wished that she didn't need to depend on us. For me, changing roles from daughter to caretaker was incredibly challenging. I must admit there are plenty of other things that I would rather do. To say I didn't sign up for this would have to be the understatement of the year. I have to remind myself that it's not all about me.

Thinking back, perhaps that is why Mother would on occasion abruptly start crying. And I do mean crocodile-tears crying. Seeing Mother cry nearly broke my heart. I would comfort her and beg her to stop crying. There is nothing worse than seeing someone you love cry, especially when they don't have the ability to tell you why they are crying so that you at least have a chance to make things better. I would hold Mother for a few minutes and wipe away her tears. Of course, I would ask, "Why are you crying?" half hoping for an explanation. She would never respond, but she didn't have to. I would be crying too if I were in her shoes. What else could she do? What could any of us do? I would hug Mother and tell her that I loved her, realizing that it had been a while since I had done both. I felt bad for denying Mother the gift of feeling loved, feeling human, feeling like a person, and feeling cared for. Maybe her suffering is my suffering. I prayed then and I pray now for Mother's suffering to be over. I pray for Mother to be free of Alzheimer's by any means possible.

At first, the thief called Alzheimer's just takes a little, making its victims forgetful. But things get worse—scary worse. The thief comes back for more, confusing its helpless victims: they have no idea what you're talking about and think you're the crazy one. Then the thief is bodacious enough to rob its victims of their independence, their dignity, and their spirit. What is worse, the family and friends are aware of what is happening, but there is absolutely nothing anyone can do about it. Everyone is helpless.

Chapter 10

I Remember ... *the Decision*

I know deep down in my soul that this is not how Mother envisioned her life unfolding. She worked like a dog for us, and just when she was finally at a good place in life and beginning to enjoy the fruits of her labor, everything changed for her and for all of us. Prior to being diagnosed with Alzheimer's, Mother was able to live life on her terms. If she wanted to work, she worked. If she wanted to travel, she traveled. If she wanted to sit at the casino all day and play slots, then that is what she did.

And she took her sweet time in everything she decided to do. If she was making an outfit or a wedding dress for someone, she would make sure every detail was as it was supposed to be. For some things I wouldn't put in the time and effort to do it right, but Mother made it a point to not cut corners. Maybe that is why so many people hired Mother as their personal seamstress. There was definitely no rushing her. If I had to try on a piece of clothing one more time, I don't know what I would do. But Mother was persistent. She said, "If I'm going to make it, it's going to be right!"

I've never won an argument with Mother, nor have I been brave enough to try. When you have a difference of opinion with friends or acquaintances, it's only natural to pull out every bargaining chip or persuasive tool you know to get your point across. But when it is your mother on the other side of the argument, she somehow has a cunning path to the core of your heart with the ability to cause you to spend many sleepless nights. The fact is, Mother had a way of always being right, even when she was dead wrong.

As Mother's symptoms progressed and she became more forgetful, I continued to pick her up and we went to choir practice together. Eventually,

Mother had to relinquish her role as president of the mass choir, but she was still able to sit next to me in the choir stand and participate. For the most part, she remembered all of the old songs we sang and was productive.

On the way to church, we would stop to pick up one of our church members, Ms. Lila, to give her a ride. The short drive from Ms. Lila's home to church began to feel increasingly long and awkward. As polite as Mother was prior to her diagnosis is as polite as she was afterwards. However, Mother could not save herself from herself, and we had to run interference on many occasions.

One day when we pulled in front of Ms. Lila home to pick her up, she came out to the car, opened the door to get in, and said hello to everyone. Mother was the first one to open her mouth and replied, "How are you doing, Lila?" Ms. Lila replied, "I'm fine. How are you?" There was no telling what was going to come out, but Mother replied, "I'm fine; thanks for asking."

I should have known that Mother would continue running her mouth, as she had the gift of gab even in her current state. Before I could interject, she asked Ms. Lila how her mother was doing. This would not have been inappropriate except for the fact that Ms. Lila's mother had recently passed away. I heard myself gasp but quickly recovered and said, "Mother, Ms. Lila's mother died." Mother said, "Oh, I forgot," and Ms. Lila said, "That's OK. She can't help it." I drove along to church and turned the radio up in hopes of grabbing Mother's attention while gospel music played in the background. The one mile trip to church felt like it would never end. We finally made it to the church parking lot, and I parked the car. As

Ms. Lila got out of the car, Mother perked up and blurted out, "Tell your mother I asked about her."

To say I cringed is an understatement. I melted inside while shaking my head apologetically. Ms. Lila barked back, "I told you my momma is dead." Mother said, "Oh, I forgot." After Ms. Lila got far enough away from the car, I looked sternly at Mother and said to her, "Quit asking her about her mother. Her mother is dead." Mother smirked at me and nodded as if to imply she got the message.

We went into church, where the three of us sang in the choir. The choir sounded particularly good that day. Mother and I sat next to one another as we sang so I could keep one eye trained on her. We made it through the service without any major hiccups. On the drive home from church, we dropped off Ms. Lila first. The sun was bright, and everyone was quiet. I was enjoying the serenity as we rode along. We arrived at Ms. Lila's home, and she jumped out of the car and thanked me for dropping her off. As we drove off and before I could raise the window fast enough, Mother stuck her head out of the window and yelled, "Tell your mother I asked about her."

I didn't stop but kept my attention on the road. I didn't want to acknowledge what just happened, but something got the best of me. When we came to a stoplight, I slowly turned and just looked at Mother. She said with attitude, "Why in the hell are you looking at me for?" For this I had nothing. "No reason," I replied and proceeded to drive her home. When I told Felicia about what Mother said to Ms. Lila, we both had to laugh. It so wasn't funny, but it was also very funny. We simply had to laugh because we couldn't make this stuff up.

I had to tell myself that it was OK to laugh and to be happy. That is what Mother would want for herself and especially for us. It's hard sometimes to be in such a good place, knowing full well that Mother is in a horrific state of health. Denial quickly fades when it is written all over your face in the form of tears in the shower, awkward smirks when people just stare to see what she will do or say next, and just plain old grief. Not often am I at a loss for words but watching Mother slowly deteriorating right before my eyes has to be the ultimate test of strength and faith. I get weak sometimes, but when I need to find encouragement and strength, I have to lean more on Him. I am reminded that God is in control when I read in his Word Psalm 23:

> 1 The LORD is my shepherd; I shall not want.
> 2 He maketh me to lie down in green pastures: he leadeth me beside the still waters.
> 3 He restoreth my soul: he leadeth me in the paths of righteousness for his name's sake.
> 4 Yea, though I walk through the valley of the shadow of death, I will fear no evil: for thou art with me; thy rod and thy staff they comfort me.
> 5 Thou preparest a table before me in the presence of mine enemies: thou anointest my head with oil; my cup runneth over.
> 6 Surely goodness and mercy shall follow me all the days of my life: and I will dwell in the house of the LORD forever.

Verse six is what I find myself repeating often as I watch Mother's mind disappearing into a small hole like sand sifting through an hourglass. When the hourglass is empty, much like our world sometimes, it is comforting to know that someone is able and will flip things upside down to start anew. But with Alzheimer's each piece of the person that goes away is forever lost and you can't flip things around or start over. You are simply left with a shell of the person, a shell of what once was. Surely, one of these days, Mother will escape this life sentence of doom and gloom and His revelation of mercy and peace shall endure.

  As Mother continued on her downward spiral resulting from the effects of Alzheimer's, it became abundantly clear that she required more care than we were able or willing to give. It's hard to put it like that, but that is simply the way it was. As Mother's dementia progressed, the wear and tear on Felicia took its toll. She was burned out and was going downhill fast. We did too little too late to help the caregiver, and Felicia and Mother suffered for it. I strongly believe that Felicia had several untreated or self-treated nervous breakdowns, especially over the last few years while taking care of Mother. At one point, I was more afraid for Felicia than I was for Mother. My heart ached for them both. They had such interdependence and reliance on one another that as Mother declined more, so did Felicia. They each lost their companion in one another. I don't think anyone could be fully prepared for the changes they were forced to endure. Although neither of them had a vote, they both were drastically impacted by what was happening around them and to them. The normal mother-daughter relationship no longer existed as it once did. It came to a point where they could no longer care for themselves, let alone one another.

Even though we helped out on the weekends to give Felicia a break, it got to the point where the weekends weren't long enough or frequent enough. Felicia was overwhelmed. Even so, she was still reluctant to allow others to help except how and when she wanted. I guess this was the only way she could be in control because Lord knows there was not much in her life where she had any control at all. There came a point when Felicia finally realized that she needed more time for herself and allowed Mother to start attending adult day care.

We were hoping that Felicia would use this time to sleep, rest, and relax. However, I think Felicia was past the point of no return, and she started drinking alcohol to help her cope. I suspect she was trying to drink her pain away. It pained me to see her in such a mess. I felt helpless. I'm sure she felt trapped.

I was able to relax some now that Mother was spending time at the adult day center. But even after Mother was picked up to go to the adult day care center, Felicia would go to the center to check on her. I tried telling Felicia to use that time for herself, but honestly I don't think she knew what to do with herself. Her life had been taking care of Mother for such a long time that she looked lost. She couldn't figure out what to do. Occasionally, she called me to rant, and I could tell by her tone that she was a little tipsy. She acknowledged when she had been drinking, and I must admit I couldn't blame her. With everything that was happening around her and to her, I thought the least she could do was to have a drink or two. Luckily, I lived close by and could drop by and check on her and Mother just to make sure they were OK. They were not good by any means, but at least they were OK.

It wasn't uncommon for Felicia to call me and Mike to come help her get Mother out of the car after going to an appointment. Mike would jump in the car and drive over to get Mother inside the house. Once he got Mother inside the house and left, I had no idea what was going on inside the home they shared.

As a family, we had been struggling with the long-term care discussion. We had gone back and forth. One day it was yes, the next day it was no. There was a lot of turmoil, because we knew that this was something Mother never would want. But there comes a point when you have to do not so much what is desired but what is best. Mother was consistently demanding more and more time and attention than we could not adequately provide.

We received a frantic call one Wednesday evening. It was Felicia on the phone saying that Mother had "fell out." When I asked what she meant, Felicia said, "She just fell out, and I can't get her up." I asked, "Did you call 911?" Felicia said yes and the ambulance was there now. I told Felicia to have the ambulance take Mother to the hospital and we would meet them in the emergency department.

Mike and I hurriedly drove to the hospital to meet up with Felicia, who was sitting with Mother in a cold and dark emergency room. Mother lay quietly on the stretcher with a couple of warmed blankets wrapped around her so much so that she looked like a mummy. She was connected to several monitors, and I could tell that her vital signs were stable. Of course, now she looked as if nothing ever happened. Both the nurse and the doctor tried to get as much information out of Mother as they possibly could, but it was futile. We were able to provide the answers to their questions and awaited the test results.

Within an hour or so, my siblings and I were all standing around Mother's stretcher awaiting the doctor's opinion. They initially were going to send Mother back home since she was in her usual state of health. But since this was not the first episode of this type, they decided to admit her for observation to determine why she had so many fainting episodes. Mother frequently had these episodes where she would be fine one minute and the next minute she would fall limp. Now, these episodes were occurring more frequently and lasting longer. While we waited for her to be admitted to the hospital, everyone was now present so we stepped outside to address a topic we had previously tried to talk about. Now we had no choice. It was time to make some hard decisions about Mother's care, the care she needed but was not getting.

We had previously discussed alternative care options. None of us liked or wanted any of the options. Things were a bit different now. Mother needed around-the-clock care, and it was time to explore what was best for her. Felicia really struggled with even discussing placing Mother in a long-term care facility. On more than one occasion, she said, "How could you do this to your own mother?" and "She never wanted to be in a nursing home." It was awful. Of course, none of us wanted to be in this position, yet here we were. We had to do what was best for Mother. It was the hardest decision we have ever had to make. We had tried every option, but the situation was getting out of hand.

While Mother was in the hospital, we took turns visiting her so that she wouldn't be alone. I was given the job of touring long-term care facilities to see about a possible good fit for Mother. Just when I found the perfect place, Felicia changed her mind. Since she held the power of attorney, she felt like she had the final say on everything. I kindly told her that Mother had the opportunity to get good care in an excellent facility and that this opportunity may not present at a later date. Everyone was on board except Felicia, who was a total mess. At that point, I could only think about what was best for Mother. I know it was difficult for Felicia. Heck, it was difficult for all of us. Through many outbursts and much soul searching, Felicia finally relented and agreed to a nice facility I found. Shonie was living out of state and didn't have much of a say in the matter.

When Mother was discharged from the hospital, she was transferred to Eden Gate Nursing Center. We were lucky they had a bed available for Mother, as this facility is in high demand. It is nestled in a nice part of town surrounded by a rolling lawn among modest, regal family compounds. Felicia and I arrived at Eden Gate ahead of Mother to help get her room ready for arrival. When we got there, we found that Mother was assigned to a semi-private room. Her bed was located just inside the door, next to the bathroom but furthest from the window. I could see why the beds next to the window are considered prime as the view was a nice distraction from the bland, pale walls that lined the quaint room.

Of course, the bed next to the window was already occupied by a lady, Mrs. Milton, who seemed none too pleased to be getting a new roommate. We said hello to her and attempted to make Mother's side of the room warm and cozy. We had our work cut out for us. It seemed like nothing we did made the room more inviting or comforting. After we had done all that we could do, we waited for Mother to arrive.

When Mother finally arrived by ambulance, we were there to greet her and make sure everything went smoothly with the transition. I'm pretty sure she knew something was different. We helped get Mother tucked into bed, as it was after seven o'clock in the evening and she was still weak from being hospitalized. The admission nurse came in to check her in and to ask us a few questions. We provided all of our contact numbers. Once the business had been taken care of and the papers signed, we directed our attention to Mother. Felicia and I made small talk with her and showered her with hugs and kisses. We explained to her that this was her new room. We also introduced Mother to her new roommate. Mrs. Milton said hello but didn't turn our way. After more small talk, Mother finally drifted off to sleep.

Felicia and I felt this was a good time to leave, as it appeared Mother was resting quietly. We both walked down the hallway and out the front door of Eden Gate, not saying much to one another. Felicia got in her car, I got into mine, and we drove off in separate directions. It was a long drive home. I questioned if we were making the right decision and if we had explored all options. Of course it was, and of course we had. I didn't realize how draining all of this would be. I had a plethora of emotions swarming inside my head. I didn't know whether to laugh or cry, so when I got home I did both.

I remember how difficult it was to come to the conclusion that placing Mother in Eden Gate was something that we had to do. Everyone struggled with whether or not we were making the right decision. There is no right or wrong choice in the matter. Felicia had a particularly difficult time. None of us wanted this for Mother, but she really made this hard time even more difficult with her outbursts and accusations. We let her have her say, but in the end I think she even realized that we had exhausted our humble resources. It had been long past the time for Mother to get the around-the-clock care she needed and deserved. Still, this was one of the toughest decisions we would ever have to make.

This journey had long ago taken us to many new highs and lows that even I began to question why or how this was happening to Mother and to us. Soon after we realized how ugly Alzheimer's is and can be, I informed Mike that if I ended up like that, it was OK to let me go. We all knew "like that" meant like Mother. It's just plain easier and perhaps a bit selfish not to go through all of the ugliness and experience what has happened to our family.

This thief I speak of has the audacity to strike in broad daylight, yet no one can seem to catch it. The thief has robbed Mother of a life of independence where she once danced to the beat of her own drum. Now that drum beats her. The thief has robbed Mother of her once vibrant, life-of-the party personality that made you want to gravitate to her. Now people are more inclined to run in the opposite direction. The thief has robbed her of dignity, which no one would question because she walked the walk. Now, she can barely walk and rarely ever talks. This thief is ruthless.

Chapter 11

I Remember ... *the Visit*

It was a frantic Friday for me. I couldn't wait for the day to start so the weekend could begin. One of the many things on my to-do list was a visit with Mother. It seemed that with so much going on in my life, I found the time or made the time to do everything else, so I needed to fit into my busy schedule some quality time with Mother. She had settled nicely into Eden Gate and seemed to be adjusting well. It pained me to think this is where we were, but the fact is, Mother was in the best place for her at this particular time in her life. No, I didn't like it at all, but this was the hand we had been dealt.

As we quickly learned on this Alzheimer's journey, we are in control of absolutely nothing. We must learn to deal with the situation for what it is and adjust accordingly. Some days are more difficult than others. It was a long, tough battle to get Mother into Eden Gate. It's a shame we had to conform to the "system" to get Mother the care she needed due to all of the rules, regulations, and criteria for her to qualify for long-term care placement. It would have been easy if Mother were a convicted felon, because then the government would ensure that she got the medical care and, yes, long-term care she needed—at the expense of taxpayers. I would rather my tax dollars support our seniors citizens who have a real need. It's a shame that our senior citizens are not afforded these same benefits. So instead, we had to jump through hoops and prayed she met all of the vigorous guidelines for her to get the care she now needed.

I must admit that I was feeling a bit guilty, as it had been over a week since I had last visited Mother. I knew that my siblings visited her as well, but that didn't absolve me of my duty. I whizzed through work and hoped for my day to end as quickly as possible so I would have plenty of time to visit with Mother. What I thought was going to be a late-afternoon visit soon turned into an early-afternoon. I felt inclined to adjust my schedule a bit so that I could get to Eden Gate in plenty of time to discuss a few things with the administration staff. I'd had a conversation with Felicia on the previous day, and she had gotten inside of my head. Yes, I had an agenda.

    I needed to "lay eyes" on Mother, and I was also a little anxious to get a firsthand account of her condition. The conversation I'd had with Felicia the prior evening left me a bit disturbed. Felicia had said, "Mama sleeps all the time. She's always slumped over in the wheelchair." She'd said that the staff at Eden Gate had put Mother in a wheelchair because they didn't want her to fall, then she began to let it all out and said, "You see, I knew it. As soon as you put them in a nursing home…" I cut her off. "What are you trying to say, Felicia?" She replied, "Because Ma sleeps a lot, now she is going downhill."

    Now you understand why my visit to Eden Gate today was so important. I had to see for myself and reaffirm my gut feeling that Felicia overreacts and exaggerates everything concerning Mother and her care. It's not that I didn't believe her, but I surely didn't believe things were nearly as dire as she had described.

    As I drove up to Eden Gate, my mind raced back and forth as I tried to prepare myself for what I would possibly see. I eagerly walked inside and signed in as I always did. The young man at the front desk greeted me with a pleasant smile and small talk about the weather. It's was always nice to chat with him, but my thoughts were more on Mother than on the drizzle of rain outside. I walked slowly and purposefully down the long hallways of the facility to Mother's corridor. I walked pass the administrator's door. No one was inside, but I didn't care. I proceeded along the hallway to my destination. My goal was to find Mother and see for myself exactly what condition she was in.

    I turned the last corner and headed down the long hallway that separates the rehab clients from the long-term clients. Along the way, I passed the usual suspects. First, there were the two African-American females who sit in their wheelchairs and just watch who comes and goes while carefully staring you up and down. I call them "the ladies." They are always lurking around the hallway and remind me of traffic monitors. I'm guessing they are those people who are aware of everyone who comes and goes, who's doing this, and who's doing that. I sort of walk briskly when I pass them and acknowledge them with a "Good afternoon, ladies." I can feel their eyes watching me as I pass by. They reply in unison, "Good afternoon to you." I cannot fault them for anything as I know that will be me one day, where all I have to do is sit around watching to see who comes and who goes.

    The next major thoroughfare is the junction where the two wings of the floor meet right in front of the cluttered nurse's station. It is here you can find the nursing staff busy directing patients here and there, giving out medication, and working tirelessly to take care of the clients who grow to become more like their family—or, more accurately, like their children. Scattered around the nurses station, you can find anywhere from six to eight elderly clients in wheelchairs at varying cognitive and functional levels.

As I wove my way through the maze of wheelchairs, I made it a point to acknowledge the people in the wheelchairs by greeting them and attempting to respond to their questions. Sometimes, it is just a kind word or a simple head nod, but I always make it a point to take the time to give them their honor and respect. After all, they are at a point in their lives that they deserve much honor and much tolerance. As I passed the nurse's station and made the first right into the TV room, I first looked for Mrs. Ann, who had been Mother's best friend since Mother arrived at Eden Gate. Mrs. Ann also had Alzheimer's, but not as severely as Mother. I saw Mrs. Ann sitting in the chair I would have expected to have see Mother. I tried not to make too much out of it and kept searching.

When I still didn't see Mother, my mind began to race. "Where could she possibly be?" I thought. As I looked further around the large TV room, which was cluttered with more people in more wheelchairs, my eyes fixed on a figure in a corner of the fare end of the room, it was Mother. It was like looking for a lost child in a crowd. I saw Mother sitting, or rather slumped forward, in a wheelchair on the far side of the room. I immediately rushed over to her and tapped her on her shoulder. She didn't respond and appeared to be in a deep sleep. I called her name, and she still didn't respond. Even though Mother typically may or may not respond to her name specifically at times, she would respond to sound. However, this time she didn't move at all.

I tried to help her sit upright in the wheelchair, but she could only open her eyes for a few fleeting seconds and then fell forward with her eyes rolled back in her head. This was not going well. I tried everything to get her to keep her eyes open. She tried, but she couldn't even if she wanted to. I initially thought she'd had a stroke and was suffering from a neurological change—that was the nurse in me. When my nerves settled down and I took a few deep breaths, I determined that she was simply grossly over-medicated. Mother was slumped over because she couldn't hold her head up even if she wanted to. Her demeanor was much like that of a zombie. She looked totally helpless and just plain pitiful.

    I asked the nurse's aide to help me get Mother out of the wheelchair and into an upright chair. The aide said, "She's been like that all day," which was not exactly what I wanted to hear. I asked for my Mother's nurse, and the aide went to get her for me. Laura, mother's nurse, arrived and gave me an update on Mother's status that was not very encouraging. Mother was as if she were in a stupor, and she couldn't even hold her head up let alone keep her eyes open. No wonder she was in a wheelchair. She was unsteady while slumped over in the wheelchair, so even attempting to get up to walk was simply out of the question. I directed my attention to the unit manager on duty that day, Mindy, who was very eager to discuss Mother's care with me. When I asked Mindy if I could see Mother's medication list, she abruptly stated, "It is against policy for me to discuss a client's medical care with anyone except the power of attorney." I replied that I understood the policy. Since I was aware that Mother had been placed on a new medication recently, I asked Mindy to put in a call to the doctor to have Mother taken off that medication, because that was the only change that could've caused her somnolence. Mindy said that other family members had already expressed concerns about Mother's current state and that they were looking into the matter.

It pained me to see Mother in this condition. However, I hoped this was simply a minor setback on this journey. It has been just over a month since she had been at Eden Gate, and she appeared to be going downhill fast. I prayed that I was wrong. That would mean that Felicia was right, which I don't have a problem with. I'm just glad this issue was being addressed.

After discussing Mother's care with both Mindy and Laura, I felt comfortable that our concerns had been heard and were being looked into. I returned to Mother's side and just sat with her, holding her hand, caressing her face, and reassuring her—as well as myself—that everything would be alright. Although she seemed oblivious to my presence or what was going on with her, it comforted me to know I was there to care for her in this time of need. Lord knows, she definitely couldn't care for herself.

Our prayers were heard. Once Mother's medications were adjusted, she slowly but surely became more alert. The particular medication she was started on caused drowsiness, but it made Mother sleep all the time. It took about a week to notice some improvement in her level of consciousness as the medication slowly got out of her system. After about two weeks, she was back to her old self.

At Eden Gate, Mother was known for wandering all over the nursing facility. It was not a surprise to find Mother on a different wing or in someone's room exploring wherever her mind took her. Little did Mother know that, for the most part, she was merely walking around in circles. In fact, when we went to visit, there was no telling where we would find her. She just roamed around totally oblivious to her surroundings. Each day, she became more infantile than maternal. I'm not sure exactly how to describe her except as a senior citizen with the functional level of an infant. There are no words to explain, and it is difficult to comprehend.

    This is not a rosy world we live in, and sometimes there are no winners. With Alzheimer's, everyone loses.

Chapter 12

I Remember ... *the Cafe*

It had been two months since Mother transitioned to living at Eden Gate. I finally felt comfortable with saying that the rough patches were over and that this had indeed been a good decision on Mother's behalf. Mother was safe and in a good place, and that was all I cared about. If she thought she was on a leisurely walk in the park, then so be it. Who was I to deny Mother what little life she had left in her? At this point, I could not remotely imagine what went on in that head of hers. I only hoped that it was more pleasant than the face I saw staring back as I looked into her hallow eyes. I tried to make sense of things, but nothing made sense anymore.

    Just when I thought I could focus on myself for a little while and have some me time, I was interrupted by the vibration of my cellphone. It was Felicia. Right now I could only take her in small doses, so I intentionally allowed the call to go to voicemail. I would listen to her message later; I didn't feel like talking to her at that moment. I was casually doing a little housework before I planned to head out to the gym when my phone started vibrating again. It was her again. I was just about to let the call go to voicemail yet again when I figured that just maybe Felicia had something important she wanted to talk about since she had repeatedly called me in a short time span. I hesitantly answered the call. I tried to brace myself, not so much for what would come out of her mouth but for what my response may be to whatever it was she had to say. Nothing could prepare me for what came next. Our conversation went like this:

    Felicia: *"Hello. This is Felicia."*

Me: *"I know it's you."* (I really don't think she has grasped the concept that everyone has caller ID.)
Felicia: *"I'm not going to keep you too long."* (She always goes on and on about a topic that should only take a few minutes.) *"Well, you know Mama's not doing too well."*
Me: *"No, I had no idea. What exactly do you mean"?*
Felicia: *"Well, she's going downhill."* (Now she had my attention.)
Me: *"I was just with her the other day, and she seemed to be doing fine."*
Felicia: *"I need for them* (referring to the nursing staff) *to take care of my mother."*
Me: *"They are. Can you tell me what you're talking about?*
Felicia: *"Well, I don't like the clothes they put on her. The clothes don't match, and I don't want Mama looking like any old thing."*

I had to pause and take a deep breath before I responded. Was she really complaining about Mother's clothing not matching? I didn't say anything, and only allowed Felicia to express all of her concerns. After she finished, I wanted to jump through the phone and shake the living daylights out of her.

Felicia and most of my family, including myself, sometimes forget that this mother now is very different from our other mother—the mother we had before Alzheimer's. Our mother, before the thief reared its ugly head, liked things a particular way. She had originally wanted to be a hairdresser, and she had a flair for hair and makeup that she used to her advantage.

I remember how she would take hours to begin her regimen to prepare for church on Sunday mornings yet still arrive late every time. She actually would begin preparing on the night before by laying out multiple pieces of clothing that she would put together like a jigsaw puzzle, trying to imagine the perfect combination. Next, she would style her wig by teasing it so much that every strand of hair was in its proper place. As children, we were required to serve as Mother's mannequin head, where she would put her wigs on our head as she styled them. It would about kill us to be required to sit in a chair for hours as Mother took her sweet time styling her wigs. That may not seem too difficult a task, but for each of us it was pure torture. She had us trained well. We learned how to be the perfect prop for Mother to work her magic, passing the time by propping the black-and-white television at the perfect angle so that we could watch our favorite shows. No one was excluded from this ritual, not even Vance. If we dared to move our head in the wrong direction one time too many, Mother would bop us in the head with the end of her brush. It wasn't painful or harmful, just enough to redirect or attention and position.

When Sunday morning finally came, Mother would get up bright and early and begin her day with a cup of coffee laced with heavy cream and sugar. Putting on make-up was another drawn-out ordeal. Mother had a propensity to make sure every detail of how she looked and what she was wearing stood out. If Mother asked how her outfit looked and your reply was "OK," that was a sure-fire way to get Mother to be even later than she already was going to be. Mother didn't ever do, portray, or wear anything that was "OK." That response would push Mother into action, and she would start throwing clothes around and mixing up pieces to move the needle from "OK" to "amazing". Perhaps it was a change of her pumps, her lipstick color, hair style, or an accessory; you can bet that Mother would end up looking amazing.

    My attention returned to Felicia and the phone call. I calmly explained to her that not everyone puts as much time and attention into appearances as our family does. I reminded her that it really wasn't a big deal that Mother's clothes didn't match exactly how she would've preferred. I went on to tell her that as long as Mother was being taken care of, then maybe it was a good idea not to make a fuss out of what clothing she was wearing. Well, to Felicia and only to Felicia, it was a very big deal, so, to keep from causing any more friction, I kept my mouth shut. I let her vent her concerns while half-listening and half-cleaning. At this point, she was looking for something to complain about, so I let her get it all out. I knew very well that Felicia was having some issues since her roommate of several years was no longer living with her. I truly believe Felicia felt that no one would be able to care for Mother as well as she did. I just didn't want her making waves with the staff at Eden Gate. Besides, these were the people who were caring for Mother, and, from everything I saw, they were doing a pretty good job. When I had finally heard enough, I promised Felicia that I would make a visit to Eden Gate to see for myself what was really going on with Mother.

I hurried and finished my housework and then rushed to put on my gym clothes. I figured that I would make a quick visit to Eden Gate to see what Felicia was talking about and then continue on to the gym to get in a quick workout. As I was driving to Eden Gate, I couldn't get over how warm, sunny, and pleasant it was outside while my insides were in turmoil. I felt a sense of uneasiness imagining what condition I would find Mother in. I took a few minutes to appreciate the calm blue sky with small patches of thin white clouds; it reminded me of just how awesome and powerful God is.

The quiet and peacefulness allowed me to very clearly hear birds freely humming especially loud and rhythmic. It reminded me of how when Mother lost her words and songs, she simply began to hum. I remember it unnerved me to listen to her hum. My feelings stemmed from frustration and anger, but I was longing to hear Mother say something—anything. I remember saying, "Why do you keep humming—say something!" Unfortunately, the only thing Mother could do was hum as the songs and words escaped her. Although things are abundantly clearer now, it doesn't make it any easier to accept.

When I arrived at Eden Gate, before getting out of my car, I texted some friends, and we made plans to meet later in the day for happy hour. I thought my day was shaping up just fine but I needed a dose of friends and laughter.

It didn't take me long to find Mother sitting in her usual chair in the TV room. She looked perfectly fine to me. Would I have chosen the pants and sweatshirt combination she had on? Maybe not. But she looked OK, and today OK was just fine with me. I quickly returned my gaze to Mother. I'm not exactly sure what was whirling around in her head, but she appeared to be engrossed in the television show she was watching. I pulled up a chair next to her to join the group sitting in a small circle. I could sit for days and experience a full range of emotions while sitting there. Mother sat in the middle of a small group of elderly residents who were in varying stages of confusion, dementia, and decline. Sitting on the other side of Mother in the TV room was Mrs. Anna, who was Mother's partner in crime. Those two had connected as soon as Mother arrived at Eden Gate. You had Mrs. Josephine, a ninety-year-old black lady with silky gray hair, who was blind and hard of hearing. Her wheelchair kept her bound with both feet tucked in shoe boots to protect her heels. There was Mrs. Francis, an elderly white lady who appeared to have had a stroke of some sort but was able to push her wheelchair along while knocking over everything in her path. Although Mrs. Francis looked expressionless, she was able to respond appropriately and was quite a pleasure to talk with. Mr. Zachery is an African-American man who is loud and obnoxious. He entered the TV room by scooting himself along in his wheelchair using his feet. He immediately questioned what we were watching. Mr. Zachery reminded everyone that they typically watched "Dr. Phil" at that particular time. No one responded. I felt inclined to ask the group if they wanted me to change the channel, and the general consensus was "No." So Mr. Zachery abruptly exited the TV room, mumbling something on his way out.

  Promptly at 5:45 p.m., the doors to the dining hall swung opened. The residents began to file in one by one to their designated seats. A few would get lost along the way, but the staff would redirect them to where they needed to be. I allowed the residents to maneuver their way through the traffic before venturing into the dining hall. Mother was able to walk pretty well on her own. I often had to give her a boost up to her feet, but once she was up and rolling she did very well for herself. We made it over to Mother's assigned seat. Consistency with dementia patients is essential to their cognitive stability. Joining Mother at her table were Mrs. Anna, Mrs. Josephine, and Mrs. Francis. I pulled up a chair to join this lively bunch. It pays to be open for anything they may say or do. I have learned to have a keen sense of humor about their situations. I can see so much of myself in each of the ladies. I shake my head as I imagine myself sitting at a table like this one day with all of my friends around me. It's both funny and scary as hell. Although the staff was present, I felt inclined to take care of the entire table and address each of their individual needs.

 Sitting right in front of Mother was Mrs. Francis. Mrs. Francis was able to eat a regular diet, but it was just easier for her to eat most of her meal with her hands. It may sound cruel to some, but this was a way for her to maintain some independence. Mrs. Francis' responses to questions were short and to the point. She denied needing any help while making eye contact with a blank stare. I did, however, intervene when I witnessed her attempt to bring the cup of lemonade to her mouth while shaking profusely. I gently grabbed the cup to steady it and helped her get a drink. It was like watching a volcano starting to erupt and your mind telling you to do something before it erupted. Fortunately, the other ladies at the table were totally oblivious to what was going on right in front of them. The world could be falling all around them, and they would be unaware. I felt better knowing that these residents were in a great place with people who know and understand this population. Many of the staff often laughed at and with the residents—not in a mean way but in a loving and caring way. As someone once said, "If you didn't laugh some of the time, you'd be crying all of the time." That is so very sad but so very true.

To Mother's right was Mrs. Anna and to her left Mrs. Josephine, and the four of them make up the ladies table. The conversation that day went something like this:

>Mrs. Anna: *"What do y'all need me to do?"*
>Me: *"Nothing, Mrs. Anna, they will bring your food to you."*
>Mrs. Anna: *"Well, I need to do something."*
>Me: *"Why don't you have a seat and get ready to eat supper?"*
>Mrs. Anna: *"OK, I'll do that."*
>Me: *"That's a great idea."*

Mrs. Anna got her food and was ready to eat. Mrs. Anna functioned at a little higher cognitive level and was able to use her butter knife to cut up her chicken patty. This day, she was able to provide feedback appropriately and said, "This meat is tough." I must say it did look as if Mrs. Anna was struggling a bit with the chicken patty, which seemed to have been over-microwaved, thus making it tough to cut, especially with a butter knife. I watched Mrs. Anna for a few minutes to see if she would be able to manage this situation as Mother was still waiting for her food to arrive. Mother waited patiently since she was more apt to sit there and starve to death than to voice her concerns, let alone her desires. And the dinner time conversation continued:

> Mrs. Anna: "*This meat is tough.*"
> Me: "*You're doing a good job with that.*"
> Mrs. Francis: "*Where's my drink!*" (Her drink is pushed forward on the table in an effort to keep her from spilling it.)
> Mrs. Josephine: "*Y'all got your food yet?*"
> Mrs. Anna: "*Sure we have our food. Can't you see?*"
> Mrs. Josephine: "*Naw, I can't see. I'm blind.*" (I think I was the only one who heard Mrs. Josephine say she was blind, and I'm pretty sure I'm the only one who understood the implication.)
> Mrs. Anna: "*I'm sitting here eating, and you ain't got your food yet?*"
> Mrs. Josephine: "*I hope they haven't forgotten about me.*"
> Me: "*I'm sure they will bring your food soon. They're still passing out trays.*"
> Mrs. Josephine: "*I sure hope so; I'm hungry.*"

About this same time, both Mother and Mrs. Josephine got their supper trays. I was able to help Mother get her fork in her hand, and she began to feed herself. Mother has a very hearty appetite. I think some of Mother's medications cause her to eat more. Since Alzheimer's, Mother has had a tendency to grind her teeth. And I do mean grind them to the point that it sounds painful. The few front teeth that Mother has left are very crooked and protrude outward as if they could no longer take the constant grinding. When I first heard the grinding, the sound coupled with the imagery initially made me cringe. In an effort to better understand what Mother was doing, I felt her jaw while she was actively in the process of grinding to assess this idiosyncrasy. Then silly me, I would ask her not to grind her teeth, and she would reply, "I'm not grinding my teeth." And I would reply, "Of course, you are." It took many years for me to realize that you can't win an argument with a person who has dementia. This is an argument that you will lose, but the key is to lose with your character and integrity intact.

Of course, the constant grinding has caused Mother's teeth to dull and led to her having difficulty chewing her food. Mother was eventually placed on a mechanical soft diet, which was a godsend for her and for us. This special diet affords Mother the opportunity to enjoy food instead of having to work so hard with each bite. Mother was not having any problems and ate everything in front of her. When Mrs. Josephine received her tray of pureed food, the dietary aide carefully explained to her where each of the food items was placed on her tray using a clock as a reference. The aide then gently took Mrs. Josephine's hand and carefully pointed out to her where the chicken, peas, mashed potatoes, and dessert was. Mrs. Josephine commenced to eating her supper.

After all accidents had been averted and everyone had drunk their own lemonade and not their neighbor's, the meal concluded with a delicious dessert. I needed one last laugh so as I was cleaning Mother up, Mrs. Josephine said, "I didn't get my dessert." I said, "Yes Mrs. Josephine, you're eating your dessert." She said, "Oh, I am?" The aide said, "Yes, ma'am. Mrs. Josephine, I think you're trying to get another dessert." We all had a good laugh.

 It was an eye-opening opportunity to sit at the dining table and interact with these seniors, to experience life as only they do. The upside for me is that I could at any moment remove myself from the situation by walking out the front door, which is exactly what I was about to do.

 I walked Mother back into the TV room after supper so that she could watch television before it was time for her to go to bed. She sat with the other residents, and they all watched whatever channel was on at the time. It's sort of a good thing that at this point in these residents' life, if they do have an opinion about anything, they keep it to themselves for they cannot express their feelings if they wanted to. Mother and the other residents must take life as it is handed to them. Mother sat in her usual chair and quietly stared off into space. I had to look directly into Mother's eyes and almost get right up in her face to grab her gaze. In a small window of fate my eyes caught her eyes. Mother looked at me as if to say, "What are you looking at?" I reminded her that I loved her but I didn't waste any time waiting for a reply. I gathered my belongings and left Mother and Eden Gate.

 As I pulled out of the parking lot of Eden Gate, I breathed a sigh of relief that I had been able to drop by, visit with Mother, and then fly out of there like a bat out of hell. But was it really behind me? There is some guilt that I just can't seem to shake no matter how much I do, how much I give, how well I think of myself, or how hard I try to convince myself otherwise. The struggle within me is more powerful than anything anyone could inflict upon me. There are never enough visits I could ever make, never enough time I could ever give, and never enough sacrifices I could ever profess to erase the doubts of measuring up to my own expectations. That little voice in the back of my ear that whispers, "You really should be doing more" is glaringly loud and clear. And I cannot help but agree with it.

    On this day, I pushed the voice out of my head as turned up the music on the radio station in hopes of drowning it out. As I channeled my thoughts to the music playing in the background, I immediately began to feel a little better. Once I pulled up to the restaurant for happy hour with my friends, I felt much better knowing that I could drink away some of the inner turmoil that had a way of messing with my head.

    As I approached the empty seat waiting for me to occupy it, the bartender nodded. I ordered a double. She kindly asked, "What do you prefer?" And I replied, "Dealer's choice."

Chapter 13
I Remember ... *the Reflection*

Mother had a style all her own. There was the way everyone else did things, and then there was Mother's way, which was how she liked it. Mother's way was often just on the cusp of being edgy yet exciting. To say her style was a bit over the top is an understatement. From as far back as I can remember, we all watched Mother as if we were looking at a movie star getting ready for a world premiere. It was like watching a show; only mother was the show. The preparation for one of Mother's date nights was only half as entertaining as the date itself. We knew early on that when Mother talked, people listened.

Nowadays, Mother has many looks, and none of them is very flattering. The thief has not only altered her mind, but it has altered her body as well, particularly her facial features. What once was a vision of bold jaw lines and full luscious lips has morphed into an abstract glob of disjointed characteristics that are amplified by irregular, confused, and chaotic lines. If Mother could see herself now, even she would be surprised. We no longer look for our dear mother for she is no longer with us. The person who greets us when we visit Eden Gate is walking around the hallways with her gray hair pulled back starkly in a dull beige rubber band. She has lost her stance, her appearance, and the gait of a proud, independent, black woman. We attempted to keep Mother in her wig for as long as possible, but it just got to be too much for the staff to manage. I got tired of straightening Mother's wig and styling it, too. More often than not, her wig looked as if it was perched on top of her head and required constant adjusting. There is nothing worse than a crooked hairpiece. I couldn't stand the sight of looking at the shape the wig was in and felt it was past time to put the wig on the shelf and only bring it out for special occasions. So, I let Mother wear her natural hair. I had no idea this decision would cause a major ruckus in the family because not everyone liked this idea.

Mother's clothes are just that—clothes. Her clothing now consists mostly of jeans, sweaters, and tennis shoes. There came a point where we had to compromise style for comfort and safety. The staff at Eden Gate frequently comments on how pretty Mother looks in her pictures. Those were the good old days, which now seem like they were so long ago. Now, all we have are pictures to remind us of how things once were and how starkly different things had become.

I will never forget one occasion when I had Mother at the house for the weekend. I had taken her to the bathroom, and when she finished her business we stopped at the sink so that I could wash her hands. Mother never met a mirror where she didn't take the time to check herself out. Sure enough, she looked up and caught a glimpse of herself in the mirror. Instinctively, she leaned closer to the mirror as if to get a better look. She then glared into the mirror carefully and proceeded to style her wig using her fingers as a comb. While gazing at her reflection, Mother pointing to her reflection and said, "Who is that?" I looked at her reflection and then at her and said, "That is you." Mother seemed surprised by my response and stood more erect as if to understand what I said. She then put her hands on her hips and thrust her shoulders back while still gazing at herself in the mirror.

I shouldn't have been surprised by what came out of Mother's mouth next. As lucid as I had seen her in a long time, Mother said her favorite word that she seemed to hold onto during this entire Alzheimer's journey: "Shit!" She held nothing back. I wanted to laugh, but all I could do was grab her and hold her close. Suddenly, I began to laugh hysterically. Mother was looking at me as if I had lost my mind. I couldn't help myself. It was so funny because this was not just Mother blurting out a curse word. It was the way she said it that captured the essence of the moment. It was one of those long and drawn-out pronouncements like, "Shhhiiiiittt," which equated to "You have made that shit up!" I couldn't stop laughing.

Mother may not be able to say her name or my name, but she does know how things should be and probably how they once were. This was further validation that it is OK for me to feel the way I do about all of this. Why should I feel guilty? Heck, Mother didn't even recognize her own self. There are many times that we do not recognize her either.

Yes, it sucks on so many levels. I honestly feel that somehow on rare occasions some things penetrate her dura mater. I know this because Mother will occasionally respond appropriately and I can breathe a sigh of relief that she is still here with us, if only for a fleeting moment. It's all we have to hold onto. When someone asks if Mother knows who I am, I can say yes with confidence even when a part of me wants to rip the words out of their vernacular.

What kind of a question is that anyway? You would think people would know what to say and what not to say. The simple fact that many people don't have tact anymore is sad. Just about the worst possible thing you can ask the family of someone who has Alzheimer's is if their loved one knows who they are. Well, I have a news flash. I strongly believe our loved ones know who we are. We pray, and we hope against all hope, they still know us. We pray for miracles every day that probably won't come true, yet we still pray. We hang onto a hope that deep in the Alzheimer's head is a spot where our mothers, fathers, spouses, grandparents, and other loved ones with dementia can go and find some clarity. On the contrary, we pray to God that while their minds are clogged and broken to please not allow them to know or understand the world as it is for them. I still think Mother would not, in her right mind, ever want to live a life filled with such a bleak and dire outcome. No one should have to live in misery.

  I remember one day questioning what all of this was for and why bother since she didn't know any difference. The thief was at it again, this time in my head. As I entered Eden Gate for a visit. I carefully planned a test for Mother. I know I shouldn't have, but I simply couldn't help myself. I had to see for myself. As I walked into the facility, I saw her sitting across from the nurse's station along with some other residents. She clearly stood out as always, even in her Alzheimer's state. She locked her gaze on me, and I thought this was the perfect scenario. I was setting myself and Mother up for failure, but I couldn't resist the urge. I appeared to have Mother's attention, and I noted her sitting a bit more erect as if she wanted to call out to me but she couldn't. This was going perfect and I couldn't have planned it better if I tried. I decided to purposefully walk past her to see her reaction. As I walked towards her, her gaze was all over me. I walked steadily up to Mother, moving closer and closer, and then I suddenly passed right on by her. The look in her eyes screamed, "Don't you see me sitting here? I'm right here." Right then, I saw more than enough to confirm, even though Mother is not able to say my name, she most definitely knows who I am and what she is to me.

I quickly turned in my tracks and rushed over to Mother and reassured her that I never intended to upset her. I grabbed her wheelchair and pushed her to her room for a visit. We just sat together for a while. I reminded her of current news events and filled her in on what was going on at church. We had a nice visit.

As I prepared to leave, I bent down next to Mother's face and asked for a kiss. Right on queue, Mother puckered her lips and I leaned forward for my kiss. As I stood, I caught a glimpse of myself in Mother's eyes. It was as if I was looking at myself in a mirror. Only this time, I didn't recognize the image looking back at me. I blinked quickly to make sure I wasn't seeing things. When I looked closer, the image was gone. I quickly looked away and gathered my belongings to leave.

Even though Mother hasn't called me by name for over two years or responds "I don't know" when I ask her my name, I find comfort in hoping she does know me. I surely hope she at least knows how much she is loved and missed. I hate what has happened to her and to our family. I hate Alzheimer's. I so wish we could turn back the clock and do some things differently. I think about the what-ifs on a daily basis. I even lose sleep over the situation. I find solace in knowing that we all have an opportunity and a duty to right some of the wrongs that develop over a life time.

As I drifted off to sleep that night, I was again awakened by the haunting nightmare that visits me on occasion. In this particular scenario, I was on my lunch break at work. I had put my food in the microwave and had gone over to talk with some co-workers while my food cooked. Someone asked, "Where's your food?" I piped back, "It's in the dryer." Everything went quiet and still. And then deafening laughter roared as everyone got a kick out of my reply. I paused, not realizing what everyone was laughing about until I realized they were all laughing at me. I was jolted awake and in a panic. Not until I realized it was a dream, was I able to relax and eventually fall back asleep. Dreams, or rather nightmares, like these pop up more frequently than I care to mention. I can't help but fear that this nightmare will one day become reality.

Chapter 14

I Remember ... *the Change*

I think the fact that you never know how a crisis will affect you or your family on a day-to-day basis is the most troubling aspect of managing it. One day you're up; the next day you're flat on your face. One day is a good day; the next is just plain awful. One day you're laughing; the next day you're crying. And just when you think you have things figured out, something else happens that causes more angst, sorrow, turmoil and confusion.

It took a very long time for us to move into a better place and find healing and comfort as a family. As is the case for many families, we were not prepared when our crisis, in the form of Alzheimer's, came knocking at our front door. Not only did it not matter that this was something we didn't request nor were we willing to entertain a solicitous proposition. But this thief, this crisis, had the power to barge into the midst of our family like a bull in a china shop with the ability to knock over, crush to pieces and flatten everyone and everything in its path.

Out of fear, denial and helplessness, many victims of an unexpected crisis often are only able to cower, retreat or give up in hopes that the situation will simply go away. We soon found out that the more we didn't discuss the real issues, real feelings and very real desires, we slowly but surely grew further and further apart. We not only stopped talking about the important matters out of fear that someone wouldn't like what the next person said, thought or the way they looked at them, we stopped talking about everything. One by one the crisis slowly pulled each of us in a different direction and left us at odds with one another instead of in a position where we could be more effective, more understanding, more supportive and of value to one another.

Something had to give and we each had to dig deep down within ourselves. It was incumbent upon us to figure out how to make ourselves better individuals so that we could then become better family members, better community members, better employees and just plain better. The turning point for us was when we learned to deny ourselves were we able to claim the victory. Denying self is extremely difficult for most people to do, but it can be done. It takes a little discipline and a lot of self-control. Once we put others first, we found it easier to appreciate an opinion that was different than our own, value a dissimilar perspective about a situation and accept an idea or concept that we may not have agreed with. It took several discussions over several months that allowed each of us to get the things off of our chests that had prevented us from showing acceptance, support, respect and complete honesty with one another.

Now that everything was out in the open and we had a better understanding and appreciation for our individual perspectives; we were finally able to be comfortable in the same room together. So we decided to have a family get-together which we hadn't done in such a long time that I almost forgot what it was like. What better than an old-fashioned Sunday family dinner, just like we used to have. I was so excited at the thought but I must admit, I was a bit apprehensive as well. Typically, these functions would not end well but this time, I was hopeful. I began to count down the days until Sunday came so that we could get back to being a family again.

When Sunday morning arrived, I jumped out of bed and hurried on to church. After church ended, I raced to Eden Gate to pick up Mother. I was long overdue for a visit with her so it gave me great pleasure knowing I would be signing Mother out of there for the day. When I arrived, Mother was in her room with her roommate, Mrs. Milton, who was being helped to the bathroom by a resident care assistant. I waited outside the door to allow them enough time to prepare for visitors, but I was getting restless because I had a lot to do for the dinner party. At one point, another assistant, Deanna, stopped to ask why I was standing outside the door. When I explained what was going on, Deanna knocked on the door to the bathroom and walked inside to see if she could help. The resident care assistant inside the bathroom was busy trying to help Mrs. Milton but was having difficulty. While waiting for her turn to use the bathroom, Mother couldn't hold her bladder and ended up with urine all over her. Everything happened so quickly. When I saw what had occurred, I immediately offered to clean Mother up, but Deanna insisted on doing it herself.

   It was upsetting to see Mother incontinent. It was even more troubling to realize how vulnerable Mother truly is. I felt bad for thinking it, but I was glad there were people like Deanna and others to take care of people like Mother. If Mother felt ashamed or embarrassed by this incident, she didn't show it. I really don't think she realized what had transpired. It's at rare times like these I'm glad Mother doesn't appear to be aware of the behaviors that have taken over her body. She would surely be mortified if she only knew. But I wasn't going to let this or anything ruin my excitement because we had a party to get ready for.

Once Mother got cleaned up, we were finally ready to head to my house. I went to the nurse's station and signed Mother out for the day. I could feel Mother's posture relax as we walked to my car with my arm firmly grasping her waist. The farther away from Eden Gate we walked, the more relaxed she became. Once we were both strapped inside our seats, I said good-bye to Eden Gate and told Mother to wave bye, not expecting her to actually do it. On the short drive home, I did all of the talking. I wasn't exactly sure if Mother was listening or understood anything I said. I still made myself talk to her, hoping that something somewhere would align and she would have a moment of clarity.

I felt the need to hurry and get everything ready. I wanted Mother to look her best and feel her best. It was past time for Mother to have a pedicure. When we got to the house, the first thing I did was take off Mother's shoes and socks. Her feet were hideous, and I could barely stand to look at them. I went to gather my tools to give her a complete pedicure. I filled the pail with warm, soapy water for Mother to soak her feet. When I placed her foot inside the pail, she grimaced and pulled back. I checked the water again; it felt great to me, but I tend to like my water on the warm side. I thought possibly it was a bit too warm for her. I added some ice cubes to the pail of water and helped Mother place her foot snuggly inside of it. The calmness in her eyes and the relaxation of her muscles helped to verify that the water temperature was comfortable. Mother had a serious case of toe jam, and it took several rounds of foot soakings, toenail trimmings, nail scrapings and foot scrubbings to get an acceptable result. By the time we were finished, I was finished. Between Mother's pedicure and curling her hair, I was worn out.

    I sat down to rest and closed my eyes for just a few minutes. As I felt myself falling off to sleep, my head nodded which jolted me awake. I looked at the clock and realized I only had a few minutes to get myself ready before everyone was expected to arrive. Mother was napping with her head tilted forward. I tiptoed to the kitchen so I wouldn't disturb her. I couldn't wait to surprise Mother. She had no idea what we were planning for us and for her.

    I knew I would be busy getting everything in order for the party and tending to Mother so I bought prepared salads from Kroger. I changed my clothes and touched up my make-up. As I peeped out back to check on Mike, who was on the patio grilling fall-off-the-bone ribs, steaks and chicken, I heard the doorbell ring. I hurried to the front door hoping not awaken Mother. I wanted her to be surprised when she woke up and saw everyone together. One after another, everyone began to arrive carrying their casserole dishes and other goodies. Felicia made the collard greens. Shonie made the cole slaw and peach cobbler. Charlene made her famous macaroni and cheese which was more cheese than macaroni. Vance and Claire added fresh salad, hot rolls and cornbread.

    Of course with the loud noises everyone made upon their arrival, especially when they saw Mother, she gradually woke up. We all sat around the living room with Mother for a few minutes and just talked, laughed and reminisced about some of the things we did when we were younger. Everyone had a story to tell. Each story began with, "Remember when…" and finished with us laughing to the point of tears. By far, the best memories each of us had involved Mother. We hadn't laughed like that in what seemed like forever. Soon, it was time to eat. We all gathered in a circle and held hands. Vance said a prayer for the family and for the meal. After everyone said "Amen", we headed to the dining room to eat.

We let Mother sit at the head of the family table so that she could see all of her children together one more time. Everyone had an especially good time that was filled with good food, laughter and pleasant memories. It was almost too late and our family was on the verge of going our separate ways but we decided to turn things around in our favor. It was past time for us to stop acting like victims and reclaim our family from the thief that was set on stealing our love, peace, joy and happiness. The icing on the cake is that Mother got a chance to see and remember our family like she remembered her family.

And then, out of nowhere, the room got eerily quiet for a few minutes. As I was soaking in the beauty of the moment, I thought I heard Mother humming. She was humming! I had not heard Mother humming in a very long time. Slowly, everyone looked up from their plates to watch and listen while Mother quietly hummed. I saw Vance listening intently and then I heard it too. Mother was humming *"Amazing Grace"*! Instinctively, one by one, each of us slowly chimed in and sang along. The melodious sound of the singing with the humming brought tears to my eyes, but they were tears of joy, peace, love and happiness. As we sang, we prayed. As we prayed, we sang and some of us hummed. It was a beautiful end to a beautiful day. When I looked at Mother, she smiled for the first time in a very, very long time.

The next thing we knew, it was time for me to take Mother back to Eden Gate. Everyone said their goodbyes and lavished Mother with hugs and kisses. As usual, the drive back to Eden Gate was dull and quiet. We were both pretty tired. As I drove up to the unloading area in front of Eden Gate, I casually looked over at Mother and said, "We're here!" The look on her face caused me to pause. I could've sworn she knew exactly what was going on. Mother pleadingly rolled her eyes in my direction as if to say, "But why can't I stay with you!" I could only respond, "Do not look at me that way." I pretended I didn't notice, but I couldn't help but think that Mother was more aware than any of us could possibly imagine. I helped Mother back to her room and kissed her goodbye. I hurried back to my car in an effort to get as far away from Eden Gate as I could.

No matter how down and dejected I may feel at times, I am reminded there is a God. I attempt to understand what God is planning in the midst of all of this. It is obvious that our family lost the cog to the wheel. Each of us, my siblings and I, had no idea what to do. We didn't understand our roles or who fit in where. We were all over the place. Instead of banding together, we went off on our separate ways and almost destroyed everything that Mother had spent a lifetime building. It was that easy. It wasn't until we took our problems to our Heavenly Father that we were able to put on the spiritual armor and acknowledge the issues that plagued us and come together as a family to rebuild and regroup. Romans 8:28 reminds us that even though our family was in exile and on the verge of being destroyed, through it all God is still in control and able to handle every situation.

    The next morning, I sat at the kitchen table drinking on a cup of hot coffee while reading the headlines on my tablet. There wasn't any good news to read about so I decided to watch the cardinal bird dancing around the weeping willow in the back yard. I couldn't help but smile when I thought about how much fun we had the day prior at the dinner and how good Mother looked. I was in such a good mood and figured I would use the Monday holiday to relax and do nothing. We had our celebration yesterday so I decided that I was going to be lazy and eat left-overs all day long.

    I did a little cleaning and turned on the television again to see if I could find something to watch. I flicked through the channels but noting caught my eyes. Mike had gotten up earlier and gone fishing so the house was eerily quiet. It was almost too quiet. There was only my dog Maxx to keep me company, which was fine with me. I thought it may be a good idea to run to the gym and get in a quick workout. I jumped in my car and put the radio on blast while I drove down the street with my windows down, radio blaring and my hair blowing all over my head. I didn't have a care in the world.

    The parking lot at the gym was almost full in the front which surprised me so I parked my car on the side of the building. As I was walking towards the entrance, my cell phone rang. I looked down at the caller ID and saw that it was Felicia. I really didn't feel like talking at that moment but I went ahead and answered. Her voice was a bit different and what she said stunned me and stopped me dead in my tracks. As soon I said hello, Felicia replied with only, "*Mama's in the hospital!*" There was a pause.

TO BE CONTINUED

Resources

For families in crisis, contact Hopeline www.hopeline-nc.org for confidential and free counseling and resources.

For more information about Alzheimer's awareness, research, and how you can help, call your local Alzheimer's Association chapter or visit www.alz.org.

Join us in the Walk to End Alzheimer's. To find a local walk, join a team, or form a team, visit www.alz.org.

DUES

We all have **DUES** required of us. **DUES** are required in family matters, work matters, life matters, community matters, and relationship matters. If people are involved, **DUES** must be first and foremost paid to self:

> **D**o better
> **U**nderstand Better
> **E**xpect Better
> **S**erve Best

The DUES philosophy is fundamental to growth regardless of vocation; it is the foundation of development and accountability for one's self and others. Claim the victory you deserve.

Vanessa can be reached at **vkharvey@att.net**

The Ten Commandments for Families in Crisis

1. You shall not put yourself before your family. Family before You!
2. You shall not cause conflict that leads to pain, guilt, or frustration as a result of loss.
3. You shall not take the members of your family and the relationships in vain. Cherish one another and appreciate your differences.
4. Remember your family and keep fighting for healing and acceptance. Acknowledge and be respectful of all its members.
5. Honor your father, your mother, and your family.
6. You shall not cut off your family but keep the lines of communication open and free-flowing.
7. You shall not tear at the foundation of your family but uphold its sanctity and prominence above all and, when all else fails, bite your tongue.
8. You shall not steal from the oppressed, depressed, or stressed but look for avenues that lead to peace, love, joy, faith, and happiness.
9. You shall not say harmful or hurtful things to the people you love. We are all hurting. We need to comfort and support one another.
10. You shall not hide your feelings. Open communication is key to successfully keeping the family engaged and intact in the midst of a crisis.

Made in the USA
Lexington, KY
14 July 2017